# THE HOW TO HERB BOOK

*Let's Remedy The Situation*

by

## Velma J. Keith

and

## Monteen Gordon

Published by

Mayfield Publications
P.O. Box 157
Pleasant Grove, Utah 84062

No statement or part of this book is intended to diagnose or prescribe or take the place of a physician. The material in this book is presented for your information only. It is our feeling that it is your responsibility, obligation, and privilege to gain knowledge, wisdom and prudence and learn about your own body that you may get and keep your body well.

# FOREWORD

I wish to congratulate Velma Keith and Monteen Gordon, who produced *The How To Herb Book*. It carries an intense interest factor. The depth of research is one of the best I have read. It has a great amount of accurate, positive information that could be of benefit to any individual or family. I would again say congratulations to the authors, as they have made a significant contribution to the health field for all of us. I recommend it for everyone's library of health and literature.

Stan Malstrom

# ABOUT THE AUTHORS

Velma began her odyssey into herbs at the suggestion of an enlightened medical doctor. He, aware of her sensitivity to medication, thought she might have some success with herbs. Although many of the remedies sounded strange to her at first, she had successful results.

After a difficult pregnancy, which included hypoglycemia and depression, Monteen couldn't find sufficient answers from traditional sources. This health need gradually led her to the study of herbs, vitamins, and minerals.

**THE HOW TO HERB BOOK** is the culmination of years of study, research, and the successful use of herbs by Monteen and Velma. They have both lectured, originated their own remedies and combinations, and have been able to effectively care for their own health problems and those of their families with herbs and natural methods. They desire *you* to be able to remedy the situation.

# SPECIAL THANKS

To Stan Malstrom N.D., M.T., to whom we owe our healthy lives.
To our husbands and families without whose patience and love this book would not have been possible.
And to Helen DeGroff, Kenneth Hansen D.C., Beth Marlow, Lorraine Baker, Garry Smith N.D., H.M.D., Cyndee Holland, Diane Bjoarnson, Helen Beaman, LeArta and Clark Moulton, and Arline Heaton.

# TABLE OF CONTENTS

# INTRODUCTION

## Purpose and How to Use This Book

**Purpose:**

1. To help you gain knowledge and more confidence in using herbs with your family.
2. To put information in an easy, concise, textbook form.

**How To Use This Book:**

1. This book was written in an order to have information build upon information. We suggest you start with Chapter 1 and go to the end for the first reading. Then as time and need permits you may want to reread many sections of this book in whatever order you desire.

2. It is impossible because of space to put everything everyplace so we will refer you to other chapters and sections of the book for additional information. You should be willing to consider yourself a researcher and read these additional sections until you know the information you need.

3. When you are in the Ailment chapter you should be willing to look up the individual herbs, combinations, etc. suggested under the ailments to discover in more detail why they help your particular problem. You should again be a researcher. No one should know more about your body, its problems, and how to help it than you.

4. There is a bibliography at the end of this book. As part of your researching you will want to read from many sources.

# CHAPTER 1

# *Herbs*

Herbs have been used by man as food and as medicine for centuries. Herbs are natural, not instant. They work with the body, not against it, in strengthening and building the body gradually so the body itself is stronger. Herbs can be compared with food; they feed the body. Just as with food, herbs need to be used with wisdom and knowledge and not indiscriminately.

There are herbs that are infection fighters, anti-bacterial, antiseptic, hormonal, diuretic, antihistamine, laxative, antispasmodic, cardiac, digestive, nervine, relaxant, etc. Herbs perform certain functions in the body, just as certain foods contain vitamins and minerals that help certain areas of the body.

Herbs store indefinitely.They lose about 30% of their potency in the first 24 to 36 hours after picking, but are stable after that if kept in a cool, dry place.

The taste of herbs helps indicate how to use them. The mild, pleasant tasting herbs can be used freely. These are usually the tonic herbs that help every part of the body. The bitter tasting herbs are usually the medicinal herbs. These are used in times of illness or to correct certain problems. Learn about these herbs so you will have confidence in using them.

## HOW HERBS WORK IN YOUR BODY

Why Herbs? Herbs have these functions in the body; they:
1. Cleanse the body.
2. Regulate the system (body glands and functions).

  3. Are nutritional.
  4. Raise the energy level of the body.
  5. Stimulate the body's immune system.

## 1. Cleanse the Body

The body was built with safeguards and healing powers within it. When we are cut, the body starts to work trying to repair the damage. When we are invaded by an illness the body's immune system is alerted and starts to defend against the illness. Everyday waste products are gathered and eliminated from the body. The body is constantly trying to cleanse and heal itself. Herbs help, rather than interfere, with this cleansing and eliminating process. Drugs may make the system sluggish, cause allergies, kill friendly bacteria, or other worse side effects. Then the body has to deal with these as well as the disease. Herbs have no known side effects.

> "There are no known side effects from herbs used knowledgeably and wisely. Knowledge and wisdom are the key words. Herbs cannot be used indiscriminately, without knowledge, no more than food can. We must use common sense, fortified with a basic knowledge of the properties of herbs, in order to use them effectively."
>
> Stan Malstrom
> *Own Your Own Body*

## 2. Regulate the System

Besides helping the body to cleanse, the herbs also strengthen and normalize the glands. Sometimes it is surprising to find that the same herb can be used for too much hormone or for too little hormone or for decreasing or increasing the appetite. This ceases to be surprising when we understand that herbs regulate and tone the glands to return them to their normal function.

## 3. Are Nutritional

Herbs are very high in vitamins, minerals and other nutrients that nourish and build the body. (See Herb Sources under the Vitamins and Minerals) They help feed the body. Many times a weak or sick body will accept nourishment from an herb when other foods are rejected or unassimilated.

**4. Raise the energy level of the body**

Herbs stimulate the energy levels within the body so the body has increased energy to heal itself.

**5. Stimulates the body's immune system**

Herbs stimulate the immune system and promote the body's natural good bacteria.

# HERB TYPES

**Alterative-**Herbs used to change existing nutritive and excretory processes to regulate body functions.

**Analgesic-**Herbs, when taken orally, used to relieve pain.

**Anodyne-**Herbs, when applied externally, used to relieve pain.

**Antibiotic-**Herbs used to kill or stop growth of harmful micro-organisms.

**Antihydropic-**Herbs used to remove excess body fluid.

**Anti-inflammatory-**Herbs used to relieve inflammation.

**Antipyretic-**Herbs used to reduce fevers.

**Antiseptic-**Herbs used to prevent, combat and neutralize toxic bacteria.

**Antispasmodic-**Herbs used to calm spasms, cramps, or coughing.

**Antisyphilic-**Herbs used to allay venereal diseases.

**Aphrodisiac-**Herbs used to correct problems of impotency and strengthen sexual power.

**Aromatic-**Herbs that have a fragrant, spicy, taste, and stimulate the gastro-intestinal mucous membrane.

**Astringent-**Herbs used to contract tissues and halt discharges.

**Calmative-**Herbs used to calm the nervous system.

**Cardiac-**Herbs used to strengthen the heart.

**Carminative-**Herbs used to expel gas from digestive system.

**Cathartic-**Herbs used to stimulate purging from bowel.

**Cell Proliferant-**Herbs used to promote rapid new cell growth and healing.

**Cholagogue-**Herbs used to increase flow of bile into the duodenum.

**Demulcent-**Herbs that are soothing and provide a protective coating to irritated or inflamed internal areas.

**Depurant-**Blood purifiers that stimulate eliminative processes.

**Diaphoretic-**Herbs used to promote perspiration.

**Digestant-**Herbs that contain enzymes, amino acids, etc. to aid digestion of food.

**Diuretic-**Herbs used to increase urine flow.

**Emmenagogue-**Herbs used to encourage suppressed menstrual flow.

**Emetic-**Herbs used to induce vomiting.

**Emollient-**Herbs used to soften and protect external surfaces.

**Expectorant-**Herbs used to expel toxic mucus from respiratory system.

**Febrifuge-**Herbs used in reducing fevers.

**Hemostatic-**Herbs used to stop bleeding.

**Hepatic-**Herbs used to strengthen, tone liver, and increase flow of bile.

**Hormonal-**Herbs containing hormonal properties.

**Laxative-**Herbs used as mild laxative to bowels. They stimulate bile and secretions rather than acting as irritants to bowel.

**Mucilaginous-**Herbs that have an adhesive, coating, expansive property and contain soothing qualities for healing.

**Nervine-**Herbs used to heal and soothe the nerves.

**Nutritive-**Herbs that promote growth and nourishment.

**Purgative-**Herbs used to cause purging from the bowels. Usually used in combination with other herbs to control action.

**Relaxant or Sedative-**Herbs that soothe or quiet and have the property of lessening excitement, irritation, or pain.

**Stimulant-**Herbs that increase energy and activities of the body, or its parts or organs.

**Stomachic-**Herbs used to strengthen and tone stomach and increase appetite.

**Sudorific-**Herbs that stimulate or increase perspiration.

**Tonic-**Herbs that invigorate and stimulate tone and energy of the body.

**Vermicide-**Herbs used to destroy parasites or worms.

**Vermifuge-**Herbs used to expel worms.

**Vulnerary-**Herbs that promote healing of wounds.

# INDIVIDUAL HERBS

## ALFALFA

### Appetizer, Diuretic, Tonic.

The name alfalfa means "Father of all Foods." It has been called the King of plants because it is extremely rich in vitamins and minerals including iron, calcium, magnesium, phosphorus, sulfur, chlorine, sodium, potassium, silicon, and trace elements.

— good source of carotene (Vitamin A) and a little known vitamin—Vitamin K, the blood clotting vitamin which has been known to help peptic ulcers.

— has eight of the essential amino acids and the highest chlorophyll content of any plant. Note: Essential amino acids are not made by the body, but have to be supplied daily by our food or supplements.

— permits rapid assimilation of plant elements; this is one of the reasons alfalfa is used as a base in many combinations and in vitamin formulas.

— prevents tooth decay and helps rebuild decayed teeth, contains natural fluoride.

Has been used in the following:

| | | |
|---|---|---|
| Acne | Colds | Nausea |
| **Allergies** | Colon | **Nursing** |
| **Anemia** | Cramps | **Pituitary Gland** |
| **Appetite** | Diabetes | **Rheumatism** |
| **Arthritis** | **Digestion** | Skin |
| Bad Breath | Eyes | Stomach |
| Bladder | Flu-Influenza | **Tooth Decay** |
| **Blood Clotting** | **Gout** | Ulcers |
| **Agent** | **Intestinal Scrub** | Whooping Cough |
| Blood Purifier | Kidneys | |
| **Bursitis** | **Morning Sickness** | |

# ALOE VERA
## Cell Proliferant, Demulcent
## Emollient, Stomachic, Laxative, Vulnerary.

Aloe vera is one of the most popular and well-known herbs. It truly is one of the great healers. It belongs to the lili family of the succulent "aloes" not the cactus as many people believe. "Aloes" have been used for centuries; they have even been found in Egyptian tombs.

— contains a pain relieving agent and is a "Contact-healer" which means it starts healing on contact.

— excellent for burns. See remedies.

— gel is used by nursing mothers for sore nipples.

— rapidly penetrates the three layers of skin carrying nutrients to all layers.

— use juice as eyedrop to improve circulation and eyesight.

— stimulates circulation in wounded areas, which also promotes healing.

— promotes removal of dead skin and stimulates the normal growth of living cells, which help wounds to heal rapidly.

— prevents and draws out infection.

— relieves itching in chicken pox.

— expels pinworms. Drink juice for several days.

— moisturizes and improves the skin. Is put in many cosmetics and shampoos. When the product contains other natural ingredients beneficial to the skin, this is wonderful because Aloe Vera's penetrating ability helps to carry them through the three layers of skin. But if the products contain harmful additives, chemicals, or colorings, they could also be carried through the three layers of skin. Know what is in your product. **Read the label!**

Has been used in the following:

| | | |
|---|---|---|
| **Abrasions** | Callouses | Cramps, Flu |
| **Acne** | **Canker Sores** | Cuts |
| **Allergies** | **Chicken Pox,** | Deodorant |
| Arthritis | itching | **Denture Sores** |
| Baldness | **Circulation** | Diabetes |
| Bladder Infection | Colic | **Digestion** |
| Blood Purifier | **Colon Cleanser** | Diverticulitis |
| Bruises | **Colitis** | Douche |
| **Burns or scalds** | Constipation | Dysentery |
| Bursitis | Corns | |

Ear Infection,
  apply topically
Eczema
Eyes
Fever Blisters
**Flu-Influenze**
Gall Stones
**Hair Growth,**
  **promotes**
**Heartburn**
Hemorrhoids
**Herpes**
High Blood
  Pressure

**Insect Bites Stings**
Joints, Aching
Kidney Infection
Liver
Nerves
Nervous Condition
**pain**
**Pinworms**
**Poison Ivy, Oak**
**Poultice**
**Psoriasis**
Rheumatism
**Ringworm**
**Scarring**

**Skin**
**Sores**
**Sore, Ulcerated**
**Stomach aches**
Sunburns
Tapeworm
Tuberculosis
**Ulcers**
Vaginitis
**Warts**
Wrinkles

# BARBERRY
## Hepatic, Laxative, Tonic, Stomachic, Astringent

— acts on the liver, promoting the secretion of bile.
— dilates blood vessels thus lowering blood pressure.
— acts as a tonic and stomachic when taken in small doses, and a cathartic, causing diarrhea when taken in large doses.
  Has been used in the following:

Anemia
Appetite Stimulant
Bad Breath
Bladder
**Blood Pressure**
Blood Purifier
Boils
Bright's Disease
Cholera
Constipation
Diarrhea

Digestion
Flatulence
Gas
Gall Bladder
Gall Stones
Gargle
Heart
Heartburn
Itching
Kidneys
**Liver**

Mouthwash
Nephritis
Pyorrhea
Rheumatism
Ringworm
Skin
Spleen
Throat, Sore
Typhoid Fever
Yellow Jaundice

# BAYBERRY
## Astringent, Hormonal, Stimulant, Tonic

— excels in stopping profuse menstruation, especially when taken with cayenne.

— helps stop painful menstrual cramps.

— tones all the female organs; strengthens the uterus during pregnancy.

— the tea makes an excellent douche; helps with leucorrhea.

— helps to get rid of toxic mucus and growths in the female tract.

— used for hemorrhaging throughout the whole body. One of the few herbs used for hemorrhaging of the uterus. Use with cayenne. Caution: hemorrhaging from the uterus needs to be treated at the hospital.

— used as a gargle for sore throats and cankers and as a wash for soft or bleeding gums.

— used for sinus and adenoid problems.

— Eliminates catarrh throughout the whole body.

— strengthens the whole body.

Has been used in the following:

| | | |
|---|---|---|
| Acne | Dysentery | Poultice |
| Adenoids | Emetic | Ringworm |
| **Bleeding** | Enemas | Scarlet Fever |
| Blood Purifier | Fevers | Sinus |
| Boils | **Female Organs** | Stomach |
| Bronchitis | Gangrene | Throat, Sore |
| **Cankers** | Gargle | Thyroid |
| Carbuncles | Glands | Tissue Toning |
| Chills | Gums, bleeding | Ulcers |
| Cholera | Hemorrhages | **Uterus** |
| Circulation | Indigestion | **Uterine** |
| Colds | Infection | **Hemorrhage** |
| Colitis | Jaundice | Vaginal |
| Colon | Leucorrehea | Discharge |
| **Cramps, female** | Liver | Varicose Veins |
| Diarrhea | **Menstruation** | |
| Digestion | **Miscarriage** | |
| Douche | **Mucus** | |

*Case History*

S., a young woman, had started her menstrual cycle with an 11 day period. The flow was almost to the point of hemorrhaging. In two month's time, she only had about two weeks that she was not flowing. Because of the young age of the girl, it was decided by her doctor and parents to give her a few months to see if she would "straighten out" by herself.

During those few months of "straightening out," S. and her parents found Bayberry. S. was muscle tested with Bayberry; she found she needed six capsules of Bayberry a day during her period. She also took a female corrective formula all through the month. The heavy flow slowed to normal the first day and her period lasted only seven days.

In a few months, S.'s periods were lasting 4-6 days with a 29 day cycle. After a few months, she was retested and the amount of Bayberry was decreased to three capsules a day during her period.

## BEE POLLEN
## Antibiotic, Astringent, Relaxant, Stimulant, Hormonal

### Nutrition

Bee Pollen, not an herb, has been called the miracle food or super food. It is a complete, nutritionally balanced food. It contains vitamins, minerals, carbohydrates, fats, proteins, all necessary amino acids and fatty acids.

— vitamins include A, B, including folic acid and niacin, C, E, and K.

— minerals include potassium, calcium, phophorus, magnesium, zinc, silicon, iron, copper and trace minerals.

— regulates and stimulates the human system because it supplies any missing elements.

— used for convalescents because it helps increase weight and energy.

— **no need to take large amounts of bee pollen. One teaspoon (or less) a day is usually sufficient.**

### Allergies

There are two types of pollen. 1. Gymnophile—pollen that is blown in the air. 2. Entomophile—pollen that is gathered by bees, which contains a small amount of Gymnophile (air carried) pollen. Taking Bee Pollen by mouth has helped allergy sufferers to develop an immunity from pollen in the air. **Caution: when taking pollen for this reason, it is important to start with very *tiny* amounts.**

## Energy and Endurance

— used by athletes for an endurance food with excellent results.
— extremely nutritional, amino acid content is a source of energy and increases strength and endurance.
— has good effect on the heart.
— helps oxygen reach the brain and all cells.
— promotes rapid increase of blood hemoglobin to help alleviate anemia.

## Other Uses of Bee Pollen

— strengthens cappillary walls
— contains lecithin
— zinc content helps in healing wounds and bruises
— coagulative properties helps stop wound bleeding
— helps alleviate uremia-blood in urine.
— a diuretic, stimulant and has a tranquilizing effect.
— offsets effects of drugs, pollutants and toxins.
— regulates intestinal function.
— good for skin, in cosmetic products, has astringent effect.
— normal hair growth can be reduced by a deficiency of amino acids. Bee Pollen has these necessary amino acids.
  Has been used in the following:

| | | |
|---|---|---|
| **Allergies** | **Capillary walls** | Growth, re- |
| **Anemia** | Cerebral | tarded Psychosis |
| **Antibiotic** | Hemorrhage | Hair |
| **Appetite** | Coagulation | Hayfever |
| **Asthma** | **Convalescent Food** | Heart |
| Astringent | **Cosmetic** | **Hemoglobin** |
| **Athletic Food** | Debility, general | Hemorrhoids |
| Births | Digestion | High blood pressure |
| Bleeding | Depression | **Immunity effect** |
| Blisters | Diuretic | Infections, bacterial |
| Blood pressure | Eczema | Instestinal disorders |
| **Blood** | **Endurance** | Liver problems |
| Bowels, regulates | **Energy** | Longevity |
| Bruises | **Food** | Memory loss |
| Cancer inhibiting | Food assimilation | |

| | | |
|---|---|---|
| **Pregnancy** | Relaxant | Uremia |
| **Prostate** | Skin | Vitality |
| Psoriasis | Tranquilizer | Wounds |

## BLACK COHOSH
### Antispasmodic, Astringent, Diuretic, Sedative, Hormonal, Expectorant, Emmenagogue

Black Cohosh is used in many female combinations. It contains natural estrogen. Women who take synthetic estrogen have been able to switch to Black Cohosh immediately with no side effects of drug withdrawal symptoms. It has no cancer causing agent like synthetic estrogen.

— regulates menstrual flow and is used with ginger for menstrual cramps. (see remedies)

— used in uncomfortable symptoms of menopause such as hot flashes and nervousness. It usually works better for this in combination with other female herbs.

— used for nervous disorders, it is put in many nerve combinations.

— has a tonic influence on the mucous and serous tissues of the body.

— stimulates secretions of the liver, kidney, and lymph glands.

— helps break up mucus in the lungs and head, in many sinus combinations.

NOTE: Taking too much Black Cohosh may cause a headache. It will go away in a few hours but you will know that you should take less the next time or switch to a combination without Black Cohosh.

Has been used in the following:

| | | |
|---|---|---|
| Afterpain | Convlusions | Headaches |
| Arthritis | Coughs | Heart palpitations |
| Asthma | Diabetes | Hormone balance |
| Blood purifier | Diarrhea | Hysteria |
| Bowel | Digestion | **Insect bites, stings** |
| Bronchitis,chronic | Dropsy | Kidney |
| Cardiac stimulant | Epilepsy | Liver |
| **Childbirth pain** | **Estrogen** | **Menopause** |
| Cholera | Gallstones | **Menstrual cramps** |
| Circulation | High blood pressure | Muscles |

Nervous conditions
Neuralgia
Pain Paralysis
Pelvic disorders
Rheumatism

Snake bites
Spinal meningitis
Syphilis
Thyroid
Typhoid fever

Uterine problems
Whooping cough
Worms

# BLACK WALNUT
## Alterative, Antiseptic, Antisyphilitic, Astringent, Vermicide, Vermifuge.

Black Walnut is most commonly associated with killing and expelling parasites, internal and external. Black Walnut is also effective on the malaria parasite and on tapeworm.

— used for Herpes and Impetigo. Paint sores with extract and take internally.

— high in organic potassium, iodine and manganese.

— muscle and nerve food; strengthens and builds tooth enamel, contains natural fluoride.

— balances sugar levels, regulates body fluids.

— helps to burn up toxins which can then be carried out of the body by laxative herbs.

— parts used—leaves, bark and nut hulls.

Has been used in the following:

**Antiseptic**
**Athlete's foot**
  (extract)
**Boils**
Cancer
**Cankers (extract)**
**Cold sores (extract)**
Colitis
**Dandruff**
Diarrhea
**Eczema**
Electrocution
  antidote
Hair
Hemorrhoids,
  bleeding

**Herpes (Extract)**
Hoarseness
Infections
Inflammation
**Impetigo**
Leucorrhea
Lupus
**Malaria parasite**
**Mouth sores**
Nails
**Poison Ivy, oak**
**Ringworm**
**Skin rash**
**Sores, ulcerated**
Syphilis
**Tape worm**

Throat, sore
Thyroid
**Tooth enamal**
Tuberculosis
Tumors
Ulcers
**Uterus, prolapsed**
Vaginal discharge
Varicose veins
**Worms-parasites,**
  **expels**

# BLESSED THISTLE
## Emetic, Emmenagogue, Febrifuge, Hormonal, Stimulant, Tonic.

Blessed thistle or Holy Thistle is most commonly used to help female problems.
— used to enrich and increase milk in nursing mothers.
— balances female hormone problems.
— also strengthens heart and lungs.
— takes oxygen to the brain, strengthens memory.
— brings circulation to every part of the body.
— a preventative of disease.
— will cause profuse perspiration.
Has been used in the following:

| | | |
|---|---|---|
| Appetite | Fever | Memory |
| Arthritis | Flatulence-gas | **Menstrual problems** |
| Blood purifier | Gall bladder | **Nursing** |
| Cancer | Headache | Senility |
| **Circulation** | **Heart** | Spleen |
| Constipation | **Hormones** | Worms-parasites, |
| Cramps | Kidneys | expels |
| Digestion | Leucorrhea | |
| Dropsy | Liver | |
| **Female problems** | **Lungs** | |

# BLUE COHOSH
## Antispasmodic, Demulcent, Diuretic, Emmenagogue, Nervine, Stimulant.

Blue Cohosh was used by the Indians during labor to help dilate the cervix. It helps stop false labor pains. Although it has been used to start real labor, it will not start it unless it is time.
— women who have trouble with the cervix dilating during labor received good results by adding 1 to 2 capsules, three times daily of Blue Cohosh to the delivery formula, 5-6 weeks before birth.
— taking 2 capsules of Blue Cohosh as labor begins has also helped to promote an easier and more rapid birth.
— used to regulate and bring on suppressed menstrual flow.
— **a poultice has been used for an emergency remedy for allergic reactions to Bee Stings.**

— contains good amounts of potassium, calcium, iron, silicon, and phosphorus.

Has been used in the following:

Alkalizes blood
Bladder infection
Blood purifier
Bronchial mucus
**Childbirth**
Colic
Convulsions
**Cramps**
Diabetes
Dropsy
Diuretic
Epilepsy

Heart palpitations
Hiccough
High blood pressure
Hysteria
Inflammation
**Insect Bites, Stings**
Kidney
Labor
Leucorrhea
Menstrual problems
Mucus
Neuralgia

Rheumatism
Spasms
Spinal meningitis
Urinary problems
Uterine problems
(chronic)
Vaginitis
Whooping cough

# BUCKTHORN
## Diuretic, Emetic, Laxative, Purgative.

— keeps the bowels regular but is not habit forming, does not irritate the bowel. Note: Because it is a purgative it should not be taken during pregnancy.

— effective against appendicitis.

— expels worms, used to remove warts.

— when taken hot, will cause profuse perspiration.

Has been used in the following:

Appendicitis
**Bowels, regulates**
**Constipation**
**Diuretic**
Dropsy
Fever
Gall bladder

Gall stones
Gout
Hemorrhoids
Itching
Lead poisoning
Liver
Poultice

Perspiration
Rheumatism
**Warts**
**Worms-parasites,
expels.**

# BURDOCK
## Alterative, Cholagogue, Depurant, Diuretic, Laxative, Stomachic, Tonic.

— strong blood purifier and cleanser, has been used to neutralize and eliminate toxins in the system. Best when used in combination with other herbs, since it can start the body cleansing too rapidly if used by itself. *If used by itself, start with small amounts.*

— one of the best herbs for chronic skin problems. The tea makes a good wash for acne, burns and sores.

— hot fomentations help heal swellings.

— bruised leaves or tea have been used successfully for poison ivy or oak.

— relieves congestion of the lymphatic system.

— increases flow of urine, relieves pain in the bladder, and helps fight kidney and bladder infection.

— promotes perspiration, especially helpful in the case of fevers.

— good for advanced cases of arthritis. Helps reduce the swelling and deposits of joints and knuckles and breaks down calcification.

— helps move toxins out of a weak body.

— contains vitamin B3 (niacin) and vitamin C.

Has been used in the following:

| | | |
|---|---|---|
| **Acne** | Fevers | **Psoriasis** |
| **Allergies** | Gall bladder | Rheumatism |
| **Arthritis** | Glands, swollen | Sciatic nerve |
| Baldness | Gonorrhea | Scrofula |
| **Bladder infections** | Gout | Scurvey |
| **Bladder pain** | Hair loss | **Skin** |
| **Blood purifier** | Hemorrhoids | Stomach |
| **Boils** | **Herpes** | Swelling |
| **Bruises** | **Itch** | Syphilis |
| **Burns** | **Kidneys** | Tonsilitis |
| **Bursitis** | **Laxative** | Tuberculosis |
| Cancer | Leprosy | Venereal Disease |
| **Canker sore** | Liver | Weight loss |
| **Chicken pox,** | Lupus | Wounds |
| internal, external | **Lymphatic System** | |
| **Constipation** | Obesity | |
| **Eczema** | **Pimples** | |
| Endurance | **Poison Ivy, Oak** | |

# CASCARA SAGRADA
## Tonic, Laxative

The Indians called Cascara Sagrada the "Sacred Bark." It soothes the nerves and promotes sleep. It is a laxative that is safe to use during pregnancy and can be used for children. (See remedies)

— increases the secretions of the liver (bile), stomach, pancreas and lower bowel, but is not an irritant to the bowel.

— promotes peristaltic action of the bowel.

— tones the rest of the body as well as the intestines.

— one of the strongest of the herbal laxatives, but it is not a purgative. It regulates the colon and is not habit forming. It is found in many combinations for the lower bowel.

— has been used at the onset of illness or a cold to the help clean out the colon and system. (See case history)

Has been used in the following:

| | | |
|---|---|---|
| **Catarrh** | **Flatulence-gas** | **Intestines** |
| **Colon** | Gout (chronic) | **Liver** |
| **Constipation** | **Hemorrhoids** | Nerves |
| Cough | High blood | Spleen |
| Croup | pressure | **Worms-parasites,** |
| Digestion | Indigestion (chronic | **expels** |
| Dyspepsia | and mild) | Yellow Jaundice |
| **Gall bladder** | **Insomnia-sleep** | |
| **Gall stones** | | |

*Case History:*

When W. or her children started to become ill, she found that giving Cascara Sagrada before bed helped toxins start moving out through the colon and the body cleansing the next day. Often this was enough to prevent the illness. Or when the bowel movement became hard or marble-like, she gave Cascara Sagrada and the bowels became normal again. If her body started to feel sluggish, tired, or achy, Cascara helped the colon to quickly clean itself, thus eliminating toxins and waste that she felt were causing the problem.

# CATNIP
## Antispasmodic, Nervine, Relaxant

— a common ditch bank weed loved by cats.

— used effectively for fevers and to alleviate symptoms of childhood diseases.

— good for stomach gas or cramps, aids in digestion.

— used for babies and young children for colic, stomach pains, teething and fevers. Catnip and Fennel tincture is excellent because it is liquid and concentrated so a few drops are all that is needed. (See Baby Chapter.)

— helps clean out mucus in the body.

— used in enemas to bring down fever, eliminate mucus, relax the colon and ease colon cramping. Catnip enemas also help relieve the aches of flu.

— a very effective enema combination is Catnip and Garlic together in the same bag (See Herbal Enemas, Enema Chapter.) Catnip's usefulness in an enema has ben explained, with the powers of Garlic (fights infection, eliminates mucus, kills bacteria, viruses and parasites, and improves peristaltic action) the two are a powerful enema combination.

Has been used in the following:

| | | |
|---|---|---|
| **Acid stomach** | **Enema** | Morning sickness |
| **Acne** | Epilepsy | **Mumps** |
| Bronchitis | **Fevers** | Nerves |
| Bladder | **Flatulence-gas** | **Pain, relieves** |
| **Chicken Pox** | **Flu-Influenza** | **Relaxant** |
| **Childhood Diseases** | Headaches | Spasms |
| Colds | Hypoglycemia | **Stomach, upset** |
| **Colics** | Hysteria | Worms-parasites, |
| Convulsions | Kidney stones | expels |
| Diarrhea | **Measles** | |
| **Digestion** | **Miscarriage** | |

# CAYENNE-CAPSICUM
## Appetizer, Circulation, Digestant, Stimulant, Tonic

Cayenne or capsicum, one of the most important herbs, is a wonderful healer. References to it have even been found on plaques in the Egyptian tombs. It is an herb many herbalists would choose if they could only have one herb. It is found in many combinations with other herbs because it acts as a catalyst.

— nutritional as well as medicinal.

— builds up the body's resistance. High in Vitamin C, good to take at the beginning of a cold.

— one of the best general stimulants. Stimulation is the key to healing. When the body and its organs are properly stimulated, they will heal, cleanse and begin to function normally. If taken regularly it will reach every part of the body.

— improves entire circulatory system; feeds the cell structures of arteries, veins, and capillaries so they will regain elasticity.

— regulates the flow of blood so it influences the heart immediately—the frequency of the pulse is not increased but is given more power.

— normalizes blood pressure; used for both high and low blood pressure.

— taken internally for an injury to stop internal or external bleeding (see remedies.) The powder can be poured directly on an external wound to stop bleeding, fight infection and promote healing. It may feel warm but it will never cause a blister.

— used to treat shock or to keep someone from going into shock (see remedies.)

— used with lobelia for tetanus.

— used for a gargle for sorethroats and pyorrhea.

— the tincture is excellent for first-aid kits. It is an herb to keep on hand.

Has been used in the following:

| | | |
|---|---|---|
| **Arthritis** | **Circulation** | **Digestion** |
| **Asthma** | **Congestion** | Diphtheria |
| **Appetite, stimulates** | **Colds** | **Energy** |
| **Bronchitis** | **Convulsions** | Eyes |
| **Bleeding** | Coughs | Fever |
| Blood purifier | Cramps | Flatulence-gas |
| **Catalyst** | **Colon** | Gland paralysis |
| **Chills** | Diabetes | Hangover |

Hay fever
**Heart**
**Hemorrhages**
Hepatitis
**High blood pressure**
Inflammation
**Infection**
Insect Bites, Stings
Kidneys
Liniment
Liver
Lungs
**Low Blood pressure**
Mucus
**Nosebleeds**

Palsy
Pancreas
Paralysis
Parkinson's disease
Pleurisy
Pyorrhea
Respiratory system
Rheumatism
**Senility**
**Shock**
Sinus
Snake bites
Sprains
Spleen

Stimulant
Stomach
Spasms
Tetanus
**Tonsillitis**
**Throat, sore**
Tumors
Ulcers
**Varicose veins**
**Veins, elasticity**
**Wounds**
Yellow fever
Yellow jaundice

# CHAMOMILE OR CAMOMILE
## Diaphoretic, Diuretic, Emmenagogue, Hormonal, Stomachic, Nervine, Tonic.

— a good tonic. It was Mother Rabbit's remedy for Peter Rabbit when he got in Farmer McGregor's garden. She probably used it to soothe poor Peter's stomach and shattered nerves.

— soothing and relaxing to nerves, helps sleep.

— improves the appetite and aids in digestion in many stomach tea combinations.

— brings a good flow of blood to the skin surface thus inducing perspiration.

— regulates the menstrual flow.

— helps in drug withdrawal.

Has been used in the following:

**Appetite**
Asthma
Bladder
Bronchial tubes
**Circulation**
Colds
Colitis
Corns

Dandruff
**Digestion**
Diverticulitis
Dropsy
**Drug withdrawal**
Dyspepsia
Eyes, sore
Eyewash

Fever
Flatulence-gas
Flu-influenza
Gangrene
Headaches
Hemorrhoids
Hemorrhage
Hysteria

| | | |
|---|---|---|
| Insomnia | Muscle pain | Toothache |
| Kidneys | **Nerves** | Typhoid fever |
| Leg cramps | Poultice | **Uterus** |
| Measles | **Smoking, stop** | Wash, open sores |
| **Menstrual flow,** | Spleen | Worms |
| **regulates & tardy** | Stomach | Yellow jaundice |

# CHAPARRAL
## Alterative, Antibiotic, Antiseptic, Diuretic, Tonic.

— a blood purifier, has specifically been used for cancer and arthritis; contains an element which has definite anti-cancer potentials in decreasing tumors and leukemia.
— Used by the Indians for all ailments.
— Helps to heal the urethral tract, cleanse the lower bowel and tone peristaltic muscles.
— Relieves pain.
— Cleanses the lymphatic system.
— Helps to take drugs out of the system, especially LSD
— Tones the body, helps rebuild new tissue.
Has been used in the following:

| | | |
|---|---|---|
| **Acne** | Cramps | Skin |
| **Allergies** | Hair Growth, | **Tumors** |
| **Arthritis** | promotes | Venereal Disease |
| **Blood Purifier** | Hay Fever | Warts |
| Boils | Kidney | Weight loss |
| **Bursitis** | Leg Cramps | **Worms, parasites,** |
| **Cancer** | | **expels** |
| Cataracts | **Rheumatism** | |

# CHICKWEED
## Demulcent, Expectorant, Laxative.

— an edible plant, can be used as a vegetable and in green drinks. Rich in Vitamin C and in minerals, especially calcium, magnesium, and potassium.

— Contact healer both internally and externally; thus it helps with pain as it heals.

Used in poultices, ointments and lip balms. Decreases pain and swelling.

Tea can be used as an acne wash. Specifically used for skin diseases. Very soothing and healing. Can be used in a bath for sores and rashes. Used for boils and burns.

— Strengthens the stomach and bowels and has been used to stop bleeding of the stomach, bowels and lungs.

— An appetite depressant. Used in many weight loss combinations. Extra Chickweed can be added to weight loss combinations for more weight loss.

— Good blood purifier, taken internally for blood poisoning. Helps carry out toxins.

— Dissolves plaque in blood vessels.

— Dissolves fatty substances, including fatty tumors and removes them from the body.

— Has an anti-cancer agent.

Has been used in the following:

| | | |
|---|---|---|
| **Acne** | Eyes | Poultices |
| **Allergies** | **Fatty Tumors** | **Psoriasis** |
| **Appetite Depressant** | **Hayfever** | Rashes |
| **Blood Poisoning** | **Hemorrhoids-bleeding** | Respiratory |
| **Blood Purifier** | Hoarseness | Rheumatism |
| **Boils** | Itching | Scurvy |
| **Bowels** | Impotency | **Skin** |
| Bronchitis | Inflammation | **Sores** |
| **Burns** | Lungs | Stomach |
| **Cancer** | Mouth, ulcerated | Swelling |
| Circulation | **Obesity** | Testes, swollen |
| Colds | Pain | Throat, ulcerated |
| Constipation | Peritonitis | Tumors |
| Coughs | **Plague, blood** | **Weight Loss** |
| Deafness | **vessels** | **Wounds** |
| Diabetes | Pleurisy | |

# CHLOROPHYLL
## NATURE'S GREEN MAGIC

Chlorophyll is the "blood of plant life." It is the life force of plants and contains life giving nutrients that are easily assimilated by the human body. It's molecular structure is very similar to the molecular structure of the human red blood cell-hemoglobin. It has the same effect as iron and is a natural blood builder.

### Nutrition and Digestion

— helps to control and regulate calcium levels in the blood. Studies show menstrual blood has 40% more calcium in it than normal blood. Chlorophyll helps control this monthly loss of calcium.

— aids in blood sugar problems.

— lubricates ileocecal valve to keep it functioning properly.

— increases iron in milk on nursing mothers.

— excellent to use in a cleansing diet because its fluids clean the structure of the cell and its important minerals build new cell life. It has been called "liquid sunshine" because it absorbs energy from the sun.

### Cleansing & Healing of Chlorophyll

— a great natural healer and cleanser for chronic conditions internally and externally.

— stops growth and development of toxic bacteria. Disease causing bacteria find it difficult to live in the presence of chlorophyll. Counteracts toxins.

— accelerates tissue cell activity and normal re-growth of cells which helps the body heal faster.

— has been used in salves and ointments for external use.

— used as a gargle for tonsils (See Ailments.)

— inhibits the metabolic action of carcinogens (cancer causing elements.)

### Purifying Qualities of Chlorophyll

— helps purify the liver and eliminate drug deposits, old toxic material, chemical spray on food, artificial flavoring, colors and other coal tar products that may become stored in it.

— helps to get bile moving regularly.

— acts as a detergent in the body.

— has been used to remove toxic metal from children.

### Bowel

— deodorizes the bowel and entire body; a natural antiseptic to the intestinal tract.

— goes unchanged until it reaches the small intestine.

— aids in rebuilding damaged bowel tissue and helps to eliminate mucus.

— reduces acid which produces putrefaction in bowel.

— helps to keep colon healthy because it destroys toxic and disease causing bacteria.

— one teaspoon of concentrated Chlorophyll (liquid form) to 1 cup of water equals a glass of green drink.

Because the information on Chlorophyll is so abundant, it is difficult to condense it. However, one thing is clear, chlorophyll is so valuable to the body that green drinks or chlorophyll should be part of a daily regime.

Has been used in the following:

| | | |
|---|---|---|
| **Anemia** | Hemorrhoids | Pyorrhea |
| **Blood builder** | Hepatitis | Sinus |
| Blood pressure | Hemophilia | Teeth |
| **Body odors** | **Hypoglycemia** | Throat, gargle |
| **Bowels, cleanses** | Infections | Tissue repair |
| **and deodorizes** | Inflammations | Tonsilitis |
| **Breath freshner** | Insomnia | Tooth surgery |
| **Calcium, regulates** | **Iron (to organs)** | **Toxins, counteract** |
| Catarrh | **Liver** | Ulcers |
| **Deodorizer** | **Menstruation** | Vaginal douche |
| Diabetes | **Nasal douche** | Varicose veins |
| **Energy** | Nerves | Vascular system |
| Headache | **Nursing** | Wounds |
| Heart | Pain | |

# COMFREY
## Astringent, Cell Proliferant, Demulcent

Comfrey has a strong history of being used as an external application by itself or in poultices for the mending of wounds and broken bones. Comfrey has been called the "bone knitter."

It has been reported in some studies that the combined alkaloids in Comfrey have been linked to chronic hepatotoxicity and cancer in rats. These alkaloids have been found in both the root and the leaf of Comfrey, however, they are more concentrated in the root than the leaf. As always use wisdom and knowledge.

Another study by Daniel O. Noorlander using Comfrey on Streptococcus Agalactia and Staphylococcal bacteria, showed that when Comfrey extract was introduced topically to the bacteria, within 20 to 30 minutes the walls of the bacteria cells weakened and then burst, destroying the bacteria.

— contact healer (relieves pain and starts healing on contact.)

— cell proliferant (helps grows new flesh and bone.) Accelerates the healing process. The cell proliferant and active ingredient in Comfrey in called Allantoin.

— helps with pain, repairs and heals, excellent for wounds, burns, cuts and abrasions and broken bones, high in calcium.

— reduces the inflammation of pulled tendons.

— extract used topically for acne and athletes foot.

— used for female problems. Comfrey tea and extract has been used as a douche for yeast infections. Poultices applied to sore and caked breasts, help the tenderness leave very quickly.

— high in Calcium and Vitamin C. Contains carotene (Vitamin A), B12 and chlorophyll.

— when Comfrey extract was applied to mosquito bites, the itching stopped immediately and the swelling went down.

Has been used historically in the following:

| | | |
|---|---|---|
| Acne | Bowels, ulcerated | Congestion |
| Allergies | Boils | Coughs |
| Arthritis | Breasts, sore | Dandruff |
| Athlete's Foot | Bronchitis | Diaper rash |
| Baths for sores | Bruises | Diarrhea |
| Bed sores | Burns | Digestion |
| Bladder | Bursitis | Douches |
| Bleeding Gums | Cold Sores | Dysentery |

| | | |
|---|---|---|
| Eczema | Hoarseness | Rheumatism |
| **Emphysema** | **Infections** | **Skin** |
| Energy | **Inflammations** | **Sores** |
| **Female problems** | **Insect Bites, Stings** | Sprains |
| **Fomentations** | **Itching** | Stomach |
| **Fractures** | Kidneys | **Swellings** |
| Gall bladder | Leucorrhea | Tendons, pulled |
| **Gangrene** | **Lungs** | Throat |
| Gargle | **Mouthwash** | Tonsillitis |
| **Gout** | **Mucous membranes** | Tuberculosis |
| Gum infections | Mucus | Tumors |
| (extract, tea) | **Pain** | Ulcers |
| **Hay Fever** | Pleurisy | Vaginal discharge |
| Hemorrhaging | **Poultice** | **Vaginal douche** |
| Hemorrhoids | Psoriasis | **Wounds** |
| **Herpes** | Pyorrhea | **Yeast infection** |

### *Case History*

D. cut himself on the finger with an aluminum can lid. The wound was very deep, almost to the bone. He applied fresh Comfrey poultices to the wound daily. The wound healed completely in 2–3 days.

## CORNSILK
### Alterative, Anodyne, Demulcent, Diuretic

Cornsilk is good for all kinds of kidney and bladder problems including bed wetting (See Remedies) and painful urination cased by prostate gland problems.

Has been used in the following:

| | | |
|---|---|---|
| **Bladder** | **Prostate gland** | **Urination, painful** |
| **Kidney** | | |

# DAMIANA
## Aphrodisiac, Hormonal, Tonic.

— good for the reproductive organs.

— helps to balance female hormones and help with menopausal hot flashes.

— helps with sexual impotency and infertility for both male and female.

— gives energy to the limbs.

Has been used in the following:

| | | |
|---|---|---|
| Energy | **Impotency** | Parkinson's Disease |
| **Female problems** | **Infertility** | **Prostate** |
| **Hormone balance** | Menopause | **Reproductive organs** |
| **Hot flashes** | Nerves | |

# DANDELION
## Cholagogue, Depurant, Hepatic, Laxative, Stimulant, Stomachic, Tonic.

The dandelion we are talking about really is that little yellow weed in your lawn. All its parts are used—the leaves, flower and roots. It can be used fresh in green drinks and salads.

— one of the best blood purifiers and builders available.

— high in vitamins and minerals, especially calcium.

— contains all the nutritive salts for the blood. Dandelion restores and balances the blood so anemia that is caused by deficiencies of these blood salts disappears.

— the herb for low blood pressure, helps build energy and endurance.

— Overweight people when losing weight can become over acidic. These acids in the blood are destroyed by dandelion.

— one of the best liver cleansers. It increases the activity of the liver and the flow of bile into the intestines.

— it is fantastic for use in hepatitis (see ailments.)

— increases activity of the pancreas and the spleen.

— good for the female organs.

— helps open urinary passages.

— used to treat skin diseases.

Has been used in the following:

| | | |
|---|---|---|
| **Acne** | Diuretic | **Liver cleanser** |
| **Age spots** | Dropsy | Leg cramps |
| Aging | **Eczema** | **Low blood pressure** |
| **Anemia** | Endurance | Mental fatigue |
| **Appetite** | Energy | Pancreas |
| **Arthritis** | Female organs | Rheumatism |
| **Asthma** | Fevers | Scurvy |
| Bladder | Flatulence-gas | Senility |
| **Blood purifier** | Gall bladder | Skin |
| Bowel inflammation | Gall stones | Spleen |
| Bronchitis | Gout | Ulcers |
| Cancer | **Hepatitis** | Urinary tract |
| Constipation | Hypochondria | **Weight loss** |
| Cramps | Insomnia-sleep | **Yellow jaundice** |
| Diabetes | Kidney | |
| Digestion | Laxative | |

### *Case History*

A severely anemic pregnant woman took 2 Dandelion capsules 3 times a day. In less than a month her blood count came up several points. Her obstetrician stated he was pleasantly surprised because he hadn't seen it come up like that before, during a pregnancy.

Another woman had been anemic all her life before taking Dandelion. Since she started taking 2 capsules 3 times a day of Dandelion, she has had no more problems with anemia.

## DONG QUAI
### Hormonal, Tonic

The literal translation of Dong Quai means "Compelled to return" which seems to be referring to its ability to restore a woman to her normal health. Dong Quai is called the "female Ginseng." It helps to maintain a proper balance of female hormones. The Chinese consider it the Queen of all female herbs.

— has been used for men as well as women.
— strengthens all internal organs and muscles.

— has been effective in all menstrual disorders including menopausal symptoms, hot flashes, cramping, irregular menstrual cycles, backaches related to menstrual disorders.

— Used as a blood purifier, helps to increase circulation and dissolve blood clots.

— Has been used in stabilizing high blood pressure and low blood sugar.

— The Chinese claim it has the power to open blocked passageways in the body.

— Calms the nerves, has a tranquilizing effect on the central nervous system, has some antispasmodic components; gives nourishment to the brain; has been helpful in recovering from strokes.

— Has been tested clinically to overcome Vitamin E deficiency symptoms.

— Contains Vitamins A, E, and B12.

— Has been used for recovery when internal bruises and bleeding exist due to an injury or accident.

— Lubricates the intestines.

— Helps tone and strengthen conditions in the mother before and after a birth of a baby.

Has been used in the following:

| | | |
|---|---|---|
| Anemia | Constipation | Muscles, relax |
| Angina | Cramps | and strengthen |
| Antispasmodic | Dehydration | Nerves |
| Bleeding, internal | **Female Glands,** | Pain, abdominal |
| Blood Clots | **tonic** | Placenta, retained |
| Blood Purifier | Headaches, migraine | Skin, dry |
| Blood Sugar Problems | High Blood Pressure | Stomach aches |
| Brain cells | Hypoglycemia | Tonic |
| Breast Abcesses | **Intestines, lubricates** | Toothaches |
| Bruises, internal | **Menopause** | Tumors, Blood |
| **Childbirth** | **Menstrual disorders** | **Uterus, prolapsed** |
| **Circulation** | | |

# ECHINACEA
## Antibiotic, Antiseptic, Digestant, Depurative.

Echinacea is often put in combinations with other herbs. It is an excellent infection fighter and is used as a powerful natural antibiotic.

— especially good in glandular infections and problems. A good cleanser for glands and the lymphatic system.

— one of the best herbs for helping enlargement and weakness of the prostate gland.

— used in ear aches, strep throat, lymph glands.

—effective blood purifier. Used for blood poisoning and poisonous spider and snake bites.

— used in combination with Goldenseal, Yarrow and Cayenne to form powerhouse infection fighting formula. Also combined with Myrrh in place of Goldenseal for people with Hypoglycemia.

— works well with Chickweed to help weight loss.

Has been used in the following:

| | | |
|---|---|---|
| **Acne** | **Eczema** | **Lymphatic system** |
| **Antibiotic** | **Fevers** | **Mouth sores** |
| **Antiseptic** | **Gangrene** | **Mucus** |
| Bad breath | **Gargle** | Peritonitis |
| Bladder | **Glands** | Pus formation |
| **Blood poisoning** | **Gums, sore** | **Skin** |
| **Blood purifier** | Gonorrhea | Snake bites |
| Boils | **Infections** | **Sores** |
| Cancer | Indigestion | Syphilis |
| Carbuncles | **Insect Bites, Stings** | **Tonsilitis** |
| Digestion | Kidneys | **Throat, strep** |
| Diphtheria | Leukemia | Typhoid fever |
| **Ear infection** | **Lymph glands** | **Wounds** |

# EYEBRIGHT
## Antiseptic, mild Astringent, Tonic.

— good for weak eyesight, has been known to improve vision.

— used for infections of inflammations of the eyes.

— particularly effective in combination with other herbs. An eye combination is made into a tea, strained and then used as an eyewash. This eyewash has been used for babies who have clogged tear ducts and by people with cataract problems (See remedies, Baby chapter)

Has been used in the following:

| | | |
|---|---|---|
| **Allergies** | Digestion | Hay fever |
| **Cataracts** | Earache | Headache |
| Conjunctivitis | **Eye infections** | Hoarseness |
| Coughs | **Eye strain** | Ulcers |
| Diabetes | **Glaucoma** | **Vision improvement** |

# FENNEL
## Antispasmodic, Diuretic, Emmenagogue, Stomachic.

Fennel is most commonly known as a sweet cooking spice, however, both the seed and the leaves are used for their medicinal value. Fennel is a good example of cooking with herbs to flavor food for additional nutrition as well as giving healthy benefits.

— good for children because of its mildness and sweet flavor. Marvelous for colic in small babies or for stomach aches for all ages, especially when combined in tincture form with Catnip (see Catnip or baby chapter.)

— aids digestion especially when uric acid is a problem as in gout.

— helps normalize the appetite, used to help weight loss.

— increases the flow of urine, a liver cleanser.

— the tea makes a good eye wash,

— helps in milk production.

Has been used in the following:

| | | |
|---|---|---|
| **Appetite** | Gargle | Nerves |
| **Colic** | Gout | Respiratory system |
| Convulsions | Headache. migraine | Rhuematic pain |
| Cough | Hoarseness | Sinus |
| Cramps | Insect bites, stings | Snake bites |
| **Digestion** | Intestines | Spasms |
| **Diuretic** | Kidney | Spleen |
| Emphysema | Liver | **Stomach acid** |
| Eyewash | Menstrual flow, | **Uric acid** |
| **Flatulence-gas** | tardy & suppressed | Urinary problems |
| Food poisoning | **Milk production** | Weight loss |
| Gall bladder | Mucus | Yellow jaundice |

# FENUGREEK
## Aromatic, Expectorant, Mucilaginous, Nutritive.

— known as a lung herb, the seed is the part used.
— expels mucus and phlegm from the bronchial tubes.
— soothes sore throats.
— helps the digestive system, is a lubricant for the intestines, and coats ulcers and intestinal sores.
— contains lecithin which helps to dissolve cholesterol and fatty substances.
— expels toxic waste through the lymphatic system.
— used in poultices for inflammation and wounds.
Has been used in the following:

| | | |
|---|---|---|
| **Allergies** | Gargle | Neuralgia |
| Anemia | Glands, swollen | Respiratory system |
| Arthritis | Gout pain, poultice | Sciatica |
| Bronchitis | **Headache, migraine** | Skin |
| Bruises | Hemorrhoids | Stomach |
| **Coughs** | **Intestinal inflam-** | **Throat, sore** |
| Diabetes | **mation, and ulcers.** | Toxic waste. |
| **Digestion** | **Intestinal lubricant** | expels |
| Diuretic | **Lungs** | Tumors |
| **Emphysema** | **Mucous membranes** | Vagina |
| Fever | **Mucus, expels** | Water retention |
| **Flatulence-gas** | Nerves | Wounds |

# GARLIC
## Alterative, Antibiotic, Antiseptic, Carminative, Digestant, Diuretic, Tonic, Vermifuge.

Garlic is called nature's antibiotic. It contains allicin, a natural antibiotic. 1 milligram of Allicin has a potency of 15 standard units of Penicillin. It is effective against toxic bacteria, viruses, and fungus. Garlic contains more germanium, an anti-cancer agent, than any other herb. In tests with mice and rats, garlic fed groups developed no cancer-where non-garlic fed groups developed some cancers. In Russia, garlic was found to retard tumor growth in *humans.*
— active against staphylococcus and E. coli bacteria.

— good to take for all diseases (anti-bacterial, anti-fungal, anti-viral, anti-cancer) including contagious diseases.

— protects against infection.

— has detoxifying effect on *all* the body systems.

— improves, tones, and strengthens entire physical condition. Has rejuvenating effect on all cells.

— builds endurance and energy.

— strengthens body defenses against allergens.

— has soft oils that help to emulsify plaque and loosen it from arterial walls.

— contains selenium which helps arteriosclerosis.

— strengthens blood vessels.

— equalizes blood pressure, high or low.

— has a sugar regulating factor.

— taken internally one of the most effective herbs for killing and expelling parasites.

— used in enemas. Besides being used as straight garlic enema, it is excellent to combine with Catnip for a Catnip/Garlic enema. The catnip pulls mucus, and soothes the cramping of the colon, etc. The garlic kills the germs and parasites, improves peristaltic action, and also pulls mucus. (See enemas and Catnip)

— Garlic contains protein, phosphorus, potassium, Vitamins A, B, B2, and C, Calcium, Sulfur, Selenium, Germanium, Allicin, Allicetoin I & II, Aluminum, Chlorine, Manganese, Zinc, Copper, and Iron.

Has been used in the following:

| | | |
|---|---|---|
| Allergies | **Colitis** | Insect Bites, stings |
| Anemia | **Contagious diseases** | Insomnia |
| **Antibiotic, natural** | **Coughs** | **Intestinal infections** |
| **Anti-fungus** | Cramps | Lead poisoning |
| **Anti-viral** | Diabetes | **Liver, detoxifies** |
| Arteriosclerosis | Digestion | **Lungs** |
| **Arthritis** | **Fever** | Metal poisoning |
| **Asthma** | **Flatulence-gas** | **Mucus** |
| **Blood purifier** | **Flu-influenza** | Nervine |
| **Bronchitis, chronic** | Gall bladder | **Parasitic diarrhea** |
| **Cancer** | Glands, regulates | **Pin worms** |
| **Catarrh** | Heart | **Plague, blood** |
| **Cholera** | **High blood pressure** | vessels |
| **Circulation** | Hypoglycemia | **Prostate gland** |
| **Cold** | **Infections** | Rabies |

| | | |
|---|---|---|
| Sinus | **Tumors** | **Worms-parasites,** |
| **Spinal meningitis** | Typhoid fever | **expels** |
| Stomach catarrh | Ulcers | **Yeast infections** |
| **Toothache** | **Warts** | |
| **Tuberculosis** | **Whooping Cough** | |

# GINGER
## Appetizer, Stimulant, Stomachic.

Ginger, the spice used in cooking, is used in the bathtub to promote perspiration to relieve congestion and fevers; and to help relax and relieve tired, achy muscles after over exercising.3-4 tablespoons per full bathtub (see remedies) in tepid, not hot, water.

— is great in cough syrups (see remedies) and helps relieve congestion in the sinus cavities especially when combined with cayenne.

— has cleansing effect on the kidneys and bowels.

— helps to remove excess toxins from the body.

— stimulates the circulatory system.

— helps with suppressed menstruation and is excellent for menstrual cramps (see remedies.)

Has been used in the following:

| | | |
|---|---|---|
| **Bronchitis** | Contagious diseases | Dyspepsia |
| Cholera | **Cough** | Endurance |
| **Circulation** | **Cramps, muscle** | **Energy** |
| **Colds** | **and menstrual** | **Flu-influenza** |
| Colic | Diarrhea | Sinus |
| Colitis | **Digestion** | **Throat, sore** |
| Constipation | Douches | |

# GINSENG, SIBERIAN
## Aphrodisiac, Stimulant, Stomachic, Tonic.

Ginseng is considered a cure-all in China. It is a hormonal herb that is good for both men and women since it regulates both male and female hormones. It is considered good for both mental and physical health and builds resistance to all kinds of stress.

— is especially good for men because it helps alleviate and prevent impotency.

— is non-toxic and used in preventative medicine because it strengthens the body's entire defense mechanism.

— benefits the pituitary and adrenal glands

— regulates and normalizes blood pressure and blood sugar levels.

— considered to slow the aging process.

— used with Gota Kola and Cayenne as a "pick-me-up."

Has been used in the following:

| | | |
|---|---|---|
| Acne | Constipation | Parkinson's Disease |
| Age spots | Coughs | Perspiration (hot) |
| Appetite, promotes | Digestion | **Pituitary Gland** |
| Asthma | **Endurance** | **Prostate** |
| Bleeding | **Energy** | Skin |
| Cancer | **Impotency** | Stomach |
| Colds | **Longevity** | Urinary problems |
| Congestion | Lung | |

# GOLDEN SEAL
## Antibiotic, Alterative, Diuretic, Laxative, Tonic.

— is one of the major healing herbs; considered one of the best infection fighters and contains a natural antibiotic; considered by many as a cure-all.

— lowers blood sugar and is a source of natural insulin. Any Hypoglycemic, who has trouble using it, should substitute Myrrh or add Licorice Root to the Golden Seal.

— contact healer.

— stops internal and external bleeding, and reduces swelling.

— heals mucous membranes anywhere in the body, helps eliminate all catarrh conditions even when chronic in the intestines.

— has been used for skin cancers.

— tea used for nose drops, drunk for sore esophagus, as a mouthwash for cankers and sores, pyorrhea, and combined with White Oak Bark to make a tea for a rinse after tooth extraction or oral surgery. (See Ailments) NOTE: Golden Seal is very bitter.

— in a combination used for an eye wash. Strain first.

— with Scullcap and Hops is used for spinal nerves.

— used with White Oak Bark for external and internal hemorrhoids (See Ailments.)

— taken with Cayenne, it strengthens the heart.

Has been used in the following:

| | | |
|---|---|---|
| Allergies | Eczema | Nausea |
| **Antibiotic** | Flu-influenza | Nerves |
| Appetite | Gall bladder | **Pancreas** |
| Asthma | **Gonorrhea** | **Prostate gland** |
| **Bladder infections** | **Gums, sore** | Psoriasis |
| **Bleeding** | Hay fever | Pyorrhea |
| Bowel | Heart | Respiratory |
| Bright's disease | **Hemorrhages** | Ringworm |
| **Bronchitis** | **Hemorrhoids** | Scarlet fever |
| Burns | Hoarseness | Skin |
| **Cankers** | **Infection** | **Skin cancer** |
| Catarrh | **Inflammation** | Small pox |
| **Chicken pox** | **Insulin** | **Sores** |
| Circulation | **Intestinal catarrh** | Spinal meningitis |
| **Colds** | **Kidney infection** | Spinal nerves |
| **Colitis** | Leucorrhea | Syphilis |
| Constipation | Liver | **Throat, sore** |
| **Coughs** | Malaria | **Tonsillitis** |
| **Diabetes** | **Measles** | **Tooth extraction** |
| Digestion | Membranes | **Typhoid fever** |
| Diphtheria | Menstruation | **Ulcers** |
| **Douches** | Morning sickness | Urethra |
| **Earache** | **Mouth sores** | Uterus |
| **Esophagus, sore** | **Mucus membranes** | Weight loss |
| **Eyewash** | **Nasal passages** | **Wounds** |

## GOTA KOLA
### Tonic

— called the "memory" herb. When used with Cayenne, it helps stimulate circulation to the brain.

— increases the learning ability when taken regularly.

— has been used to prevent or correct senility.

— strengthens the heart, balances the hormones and the nervous system.

— has been used to help menopausal symptoms.

— combined with Cayenne and Ginseng it is a great "pick-me-up" and memory combination.

Has been used in the following:

| | | |
|---|---|---|
| **Aging** | **Learning ability,** | Nervous breakdown |
| Blood pressure | **increases** | **Pituitary gland** |
| Brain | Longevity | **Senility** |
| **Depression** | **Memory** | Stamina |
| Energy | **Menopausal symptoms** | Vitality |
| Heart, strengthens | **Mental fatigue** | |

# HAWTHORNE
## Antihydropic, Antispasmodic, Astringent, Cardiac, Tonic.

— known as the Heart Herb; strengthens and regulates the heart; used extensively in well-known European heart remedies.

— can be used for any and all kinds of heart disorders-organic or functional. Arteriosclerosis, heart muscle inflammation, etc.

— has been combined with cayenne and garlic for heart.

— especially good for weakened heart muscle caused by age, and for insufficiency of the heart valves (angina pectoris.)

— alleviates hypertrophy (enlargement of the heart) and fibrillation of the heart.

— relaxes the blood vessels and thus lowers blood pressure.

— good for executives or anyone under stress.

— produces natural adrenalin.

Has been used in the following:

| | | |
|---|---|---|
| **Adrenals** | Energy | **Hypertrophy** |
| **Angina pectoris** | **Heart fibrillation** | Infection |
| **Arteriosclerosis** | **Heart muscles,** | Insomnia |
| **Blood pressure,** | **weak or inflamed** | Nerves |
| high or low | **Heart problems** | Stress |
| Edema | **Heart valves** | |

*Case History:*

An X-ray taken by a doctor showed that J.'s heart was enlarged and overlapping the lung. It was also very sore. She drank 1 cup Hawthorne tea regularly each day until the problem was corrected.

# HOPS
## Diuretic, Nervine, Stimulant, Stomachic, Tonic.

— best known as a relaxing nerve tonic. Problems of insomnia (sleeplessness) have been helped by hops when nothing else has.

— promotes sleep; makes a soothing sleep formula when combined with Valerian and Scullcap.

— relaxes the liver and gall ducts.

— increases the flow of bile and urine, and bowel function.

— reduces excessive sexual desire.

— increases capillary circulation and heart action.

— decreases desire for alcohol.

— reduces high fevers.

— reduces pain and inflammation.

Has been used in the following:

| | | |
|---|---|---|
| Abcesses | **Fever** | Rhuematism |
| Boils | Flatulence-gas | Sexual desire, |
| Bowels | Gonorrhea | undue |
| Bronchitis | Heart | Spasmodic conditions |
| Chest | High blood pressure | Throat, sore |
| Coughs | Inflammation | Toothache |
| Delirium tremors | **Insomnia-sleep** | Tumors |
| Digestion | Intestinal cramps | Ulcers |
| Diuretic | Mastitis | |
| Earache | **Nerves** | |

# HORSETAIL
## Diuretic

— an all-purpose herb that is good for the whole body.

— heavy in silica; strengthens fingernails and hair, especially good for split ends.

— helps body utilize and hold calcium; used in herbal calcium combinations.

— helps kidney problems, especially kidney stones.

— kills eggs of parasites and expels parasites.

— helps to dissolve tumors.

— good for eye, ear, nose, throat and glandular disorders.

Has been used in the following:

| | | |
|---|---|---|
| **Bladder** | Heart | Nosebleeds |
| Convulsions | Hemorrhage, external | Pus |
| **Diuretic** | or internal | Skin |
| Ears | **Kidneys** | Throat |
| Eyes | **Kidney stones** | Tumor, dissolves |
| Fingernails | Liver | Ulcers |
| Flatulence-gas | Mucus | **Worms-parasites,** |
| Glands | Nerves | **expels** |
| **Hair** | Nose | Yellow jaundice |

## HO SHOU-WU
### Hormonal, Tonic

Western knowledge of Ho Shou-Wu lags behind the Chinese; it is their herb for longevity and fertility.

Has been used in the following:

| | | |
|---|---|---|
| Colds | **Impotency** | Tumors |
| Diarrhea | **Longevity** | |
| Hemorrhoids | Menstrual problems | |

## JUNIPER BERRIES
### Carminative, Diuretic, Stimulant.

— used for kidneys and bladder problems; increases the flow of urine and helps elimination of passive congestion from the kidneys and bladder.

— The oils of Juniper Berries clear and heal the urinary passages. Used in many kidney combinations.

— removes waste products from the bloodstream.

— helps with diabetes and hypoglycemia. Benefits the pancreas and helps prevent or alleviate diabetes.

— aids healing of the adrenal glands.

— destroys fungi.

— strengthens brain, memory and optic nerves.

— preventative for all diseases.

— relieves congestion throughout the body resulting from heart problems.

Has been used in the following:

**Adrenals**
Allergies
Appetite, increases
Arthritis
**Bedwetting**
**Bladder**
Blood purifier
Boils
Bowel
Brain
Breath, short
Bright's disease
Colic
Colds
Consumption
Contagious diseases
Convulsions
Coughs
Cramps
**Diabetes**
Digestion

**Diuretic**
Douche
Dropsy
Flatulence-gas
**Fungi, destroys**
Gargle
Gonorrhea
Gout
Gums
Hair loss
Hay fever
Heart
**Hypoglycemia**
Insect bites, stings
Itching
**Kidneys**
**Kidney stones**
Leper sores
Leucorrhea
Memory
Mucus

**Nephritis**
Nerves, strengthens
**Optic nerves**
Pain
Palsy
Pancreas
Plague
Prostate
Rheumatism
Sciatica
Scurvy
Snake bite
Stomach
Throat, sore
**Urinary passages**
**Urinary problems**
Vaginal discharge
Worms-parasites,
  expels.

# KELP
## Antibiotic, Antiseptic, Diuretic, Hormonal, Nutritive, Tonic.

Kelp has a salty taste and is used by many people in place of salt. It has a high content of natural plant iodine, which is absorbed much more slowly and therefore more safely, than chemical iodine. Iodine is necessary for proper function of the thyroid, which is essential for proper growth, energy, and metabolism.

— abounds in calcium, chlorine, potassium, magnesium and other minerals including trace minerals.

— good for nails and hair loss.

— regulates the thyroid and pituitary glands (activates all glands of body.)

— helps to regulate body temperature; aids in chronic low body temperature.

— good for pancreas and adrenals.

— helps male and female organs, good for prostate.

— builds cell membrane.

— aids functions of digestive and endocrine systems.

— tests in Japan claim it is preventative of fetus abnormalities. Good during pregnancy because it normalizes glands and hormones and because of its high mineral content.

— helps to prevent growth of tumors.

— cleanses the body of radiation.

— acts as an antibiotic; assists the thyroid in releasing iodine into the blood stream when infection is present. Iodine fights infection. Helps prevent disease.

Has been used in the following:

| | | |
|---|---|---|
| **Acne** | **Energy** | Obesity |
| **Adrenal glands** | Eczema | **Pituitary** |
| Anemia | Goiter | **Pregnancy** |
| Arteries | **Hair loss** | Prostate |
| **Birth defects** | High blood pressure | Psoriasis |
| Bursitis | **Infection** | **Radiation, cleanses** |
| Colitis | Kidneys | **Thyroid** |
| Cramps, leg | **Menopause** | **Tumors** |
| Diabetes | **Morning sickness** | Worms-parasites, |
| **Endocrine glands** | **Nails** | expels |

# LICORICE ROOT
## Aphrodisiac, Emollient, Tonic.

Some may remember the old fashioned, hard, black licorice candy with the brown insides. Licorice Root helped flavor this candy, thus the name licorice. Because Licorice has a very sweet taste, some people prefer to take it straight and not in capsules. There are benefits in doing this—see case history.

— is a hormone herb. A source of the female hormone estrogen.

— specifically used to stimulate and regulate the adrenal glands and the pancreas. These work together because adrenalin helps control insulin.

— one of the best known herbs used for hypoglycemia.

— acts as natural cortisone or as a hormone that takes the place of cortisone.

— helps injured voice muscles, helps voice improvement, either for hoarseness or throat damage. (see case history)

— tonic for the intestinal tract, stimulates enzymes and peristaltic action.

— acts as a mild laxative.

— strengthens heart and circulatory system.

Has been used in the following:

| | | |
|---|---|---|
| **Addison's disease** | Endurance | Lungs |
| **Adrenal glands** | **Energy** | Menopause |
| Age spots | **Estrogen** | Mucous congestion |
| Arthritis | **Female problems** | Mucous membranes |
| Asthma | Fever, reduces | (inflamed) |
| Bladder | Gonorrhea | Pancreas |
| Blood purifier | Heart | Sexual stimulant |
| Bronchitis | Hemorrhoids | Stamina |
| Catarrh | **Hoarseness** | Stomach |
| **Circulatory system** | Hormone herb | Stress |
| Colds | **Hypoglycemia** | **Throat, sore** |
| Constipation | Impotency | Tonic |
| **Coughs** | Intestinal tract, | Ulcers |
| Cushing's disease | heals, lubricates | **Vitality** |
| **Diabetes** | Kidneys | **Voice** |
| Digestion | Laxative | |
| Emphysema | Longevity | |

## Case History

When R. found she had hypoglycemia, she was extremely upset. She had not used herbs up to that point in her life, but diet change alone was too slow and frustrating. She found licorice root. At first she took licorice root 3-4 times a day. By the end of six months she only took it once in the morning. (She had changed her diet also) Because she didn't know about capsulized herbs, she stirred a teaspoon of the powdered herb in a cup of water and drank it. (She called it licorice-flavored mud.) Within minutes after drinking it, her shaking would stop and by 15-20 minutes, she was able to continue normal activities.

At that time R. didn't know that licorice root would help the throat too, so an unexpected surprise was an old voice injury was greatly healed because of the constant bathing of the throat with licorice.

# LOBELIA
## Antispasmodic, Emetic, Expectorant, Nervine, Relaxant.

— one of the most potent single herbs, a powerful relaxant. The relaxing effects of Lobelia can be felt all over the whole body; they work very quickly and have a good influence on the body. *Small doses of Lobelia act as a relaxant and large doses act as an emetic.* NOTE: some people who are very sensitive or very weakened become very relaxed and sleepy by Lobelia. Lobelia can be balanced by taking it with Cayenne. There are no harmful effects. Lobelia is a marvelous herb; it is the rare person who is so sensitive to it.

— relieves spasms. Keep tincture on hand for use in convulsions. Can be rubbed on the body or drops can be put in the mouth and the body will immediately absorb it.

— rubbing Lobelia tincture or extract on the shoulders of a restless child is an excellent way to help him go to sleep (see Restlessness, Baby Chapter)

— reduces palpitations of the heart.

— especially good for croup and respiratory problems (see remedies.)

— extract is good to rub on gums of teething baby. (see remedies.)

— helps remove obstructions and congestion throughout the body, including the blood vessels. Expels mucus.

— sometimes used as an emetic to remove congestion from the stomach.

— encourages the flow of oxygenized blood.

— poultice for ringworm, bruises and insect bites, etc.

— catnip and lobelia enemas are good for mumps in males (see remedies.)

Has been used in the following:

| | | |
|---|---|---|
| **Allergies** | Boils | Circulation |
| Angina pectoris | **Bronchitis** | **Colds** |
| **Antispasmodic** | Bruises, poultice | **Colic** |
| Arthritis | Bursitis | **Congestion** |
| **Asthma** | Catarrh | **Contagious diseases** |
| **Blood vessels** | **Cankers** | **Convulsions** |
| Blood poisoning | **Chicken pox** | **Coughs** |

Cramps (extract)
**Croup**
Digestion
Earache
Emetic
**Emphysema**
Epilepsy
Erysipelas
Esophagus
Felons
Fevers
Food poisoning,
  emetic
Gonorrhea
Hay fever
**Headache**
Heart
Heart palpitations
**Hepatitis**
Hoarseness
**Hyperactivity**
Hypoglycemia
Infections
Insect bites, stings
**Insomnia-sleep**

Larnyx
Larnygitis
Liniment
Liver
Lungs
Measles
Spinal Meningitis
**Migraine headache**
**Miscarriage**
Mucous membranes
**Mumps**
**Muscle motion**
Muscles
Nephritis
**Nerves**
**Pain**
Palsy
Peritonitis
**Pleurisy**
**Pneumonia**
Poison Ivy, Oak
**Poultice**
Rabies
Relaxant
Respiratory

Rheumatic fever
Rheumatism
Ringworm
Scarlet fever
**Seizures**
Shock
**Spasms**
Sprains
St. Vitus Dance
Syphilis
**Teething**
**Tetanus**
**Toothache**
Tonsillitis
Tumor
Urinary problems
Whooping cough
Worms-parasites,
  expels
Wounds

# MARSHMALLOW
## Diuretic, Emollient, Laxative.

Marshmallow is a common, completely edible plant. I have eaten the little round "cheesies" as we called them, from the time I was a child. The leaves, stems, flowers and roots are edible, but the root is most prized for remedies. The leaves are used in poultices, teas, and green drinks.

— best known for kidney and bladder problems.

— it is mucilaginous; coats, soothes and heal inflamed areas in the body including genital and urinary areas, alimentary, respiratory and intestinal.

— heals mucous membranes.

— increases and enriches milk in nursing mothers.

— contains lime and calcium.
Has been used in the following:

| | | |
|---|---|---|
| Allergies | Dysentery | **Nerves** |
| Asthma | **Emphysema** | **Nursing, increases** |
| **Bedwetting** | Eyewash | **& enriches milk** |
| **Bladder** | Flu-influenza | **Pneumonia** |
| Bleeding | Gangrene | Respiratory |
| Boils | Gastritis | Skin |
| Bowels | Hay fever | Swellings, poultices |
| Bright's disease | Hoarseness | Throat, sore |
| Bronchitis | Inflammation | Ulcers |
| Burns | **Kidneys** | **Urinary problems** |
| Chest | **Kidney stones** | **Urine, bloody** |
| Cough | Lungs | Vaginal douche |
| Diabetes | Mucous | |
| Diarrhea | Mucous membranes | |
| Douche | Nephritis | |

### Case History

B.'s young daughter had scar tissue in her urinary passage from an urinary infection. The urinary passage had become almost closed so urination had become extremely painful. The doctor recommended surgery to correct the problem. B. wanted to try another alternative first. She gave her daughter Marshmallow and Red Raspberry tea mixed together in equal parts. Marshmallow tea is quite slimy (mucilaginous) to look at and her daughter didn't want to drink it. When mixed with Raspberry it is a pleasant drink.

She had her daughter drink a quart of this tea every day until the burning stopped. Then a cup every morning and night; finally just a cup a day. She drank this for about 18 months. The burning and pain went away completely. The girl never had to have surgery and has had no more urinary trouble.

# MULLEIN
## Antispasmodic, Astringent, Diuretic, Emolient.

— used in all respiratory problems and pulmonary diseases.
— loosens mucus and expels it out of the body.

— high in iron, magnesium, potassium and sulphur.
— calms spasms and is a natural pain killer.
— helps to reduce swelling in glandular system.
— oil or extract of mullein for eardrops.
Has been used in the following:

| | | |
|---|---|---|
| **Allergies** | Eyes | **Pulmonary diseases** |
| **Asthma** | Flu-influenza | Rashes |
| Blood-spitting | Gargle | **Respiratory** |
| Boils | **Glandular swellings** | Rheumatism, |
| Bowels, bleeding | Hayfever | inflammation |
| Breathing problems | Hemorrhage | Scrofula |
| **Bronchitis** | Hemorrhoids, | Skin |
| Bruises | fomentation | **Sinus** |
| Catarrh | **Joints, swollen,** | Sleep |
| Colic | **fomentation** | **Sores** |
| Constipation | **Lungs** | Sprains |
| **Coughs** | Mastitis | Testicles, swollen |
| **Croup** | **Mucous membrane** | Throat, malignant |
| Diarrhea | Mumps | Throat, sore |
| Dropsy | Nasal congestion | Tonsillitis |
| Dysentery | **Pain** | Toothache |
| **Earaches** | Pleurisy | Tumors |
| **Emphysema** | Pnuemonia | Ulcers |

# MYRRH
## Antibiotic, Alterative, Antiseptic, Cardiac, Disinfectant, Expectorant, Stimulant, Tonic.

Myrrh was one of the precious gifts the Three Wise Men brought to the infant Jesus. Since Biblical days, this costly spice has been highly valued and prized.
— promotes increased white corpuscles (up to four times) to fight infection.
— used with other herbs as a natural antibiotic. Sometimes used in place of goldenseal especially in cases of hypoglycemia.
— for bad breath or pyorrhea, brush teeth with powder and rinse with tea.
— cleans and heals stomach and colon. Improves waste elimination.

— gives vitality to digestive system.
— brings on suppressed menstruation.
Has been used in the following:

| | | |
|---|---|---|
| **Antibiotic** | **Emphysema** | Shock |
| **Antiseptic** | Energy | **Sinus problems** |
| **Asthma** | Flatulence-gas | **Sores, poultice** |
| Bad breath | **Gangrene** | **Stomach** |
| **Bed sores** | **Gargle** | Stomach cramps |
| Boils, poultice | **Gums** | Teeth, loose |
| Breath freshener | Healing, general | Throat, sore, |
| Bronchial diseases | Hemorrhoids | ulcerated |
| Catarrh | **Herpes** | **Toothache** |
| Colitis | **Hypoglycemia** | **Tonsillitis** |
| **Colon** | **Infection** | Tuberculosis |
| **Coughs** | **Leg ulcers** | Typhoid fever |
| **Cuts** | **Lungs** | Ulcers |
| Diarrhea | Menstruation | Uterus |
| **Digestion** | **Mouth sores** | Vaginal discharge |
| Douche | Nerves | Vitality |
| Diphtheria | **Pyorrhea** | **Wounds, poultice** |
| Eczema | Scarlet fever | |

# PAPAYA
## Digestant

Papaya contains the protein-splitting enzyme papain. It is used as a digestive aid to help us assimilate nutrients from our food. It is a delicious fruit to eat and is one of the few fruits that can be eaten with meals.

— relieves gas and sour stomach.
— used in cancer management and prevention because good enzyme actions are essential.
— has been used as a meat tenderizer. Helps break down protein.
— good for babies. Has been put in formulas to make it closer to mother's milk.
Has been used in the following:

| | | |
|---|---|---|
| Allergies | **Digestion** | **Flatulence-gas** |
| **Babies formulas** | Diverticulitis | Hemorrhage |

Meat tenderizer     **Stomach, sour**     Worms-Parasites,
Stomach ache                                    expels

# PARSLEY
## Aromatic, Diuretic, Nutritive, Tonic.

Parsley is a good example of the balance that occurs in herbs. It is a diuretic and yet it is also very rich in potassium. It can be used to replace the water retention drugs on the market since it won't deplete the body of potassium like they do.

— one of the most used remedies for kidney and bladder problems.

— good for nervous system, adrenals, assimilation and elimination. Good for digestion—used extensively in green drinks. It is very nutritious.

— helps dry up milk in lactation, alleviates afterpains, regulates the menstrual cycle. (Do not use parsley while nursing.)

— tonic for blood vessels, capillaries and arterioles.

— high in vitamins A, B and C (3 times more C than citrus.)

— Increases body's resistance to all diseases. Vitamin A is one of the vitamins that stimulates the body's immune system.

— cancer preventative—cancer cannot live in blood that is high in potassium. Vitamin A also fights cancer.

— contains lots of minerals, especially potassium and iron. Has more iron than any other green vegetable.

— high in chlorophyll.

Has been used in the following:

| | | |
|---|---|---|
| **Adrenal glands** | **Cancer preventative** | Gall bladder |
| Allergies | Capillaries | Gall stones |
| Appetite, stimulates | Coughs | Gonorrhea |
| Arterioles | Digestion | Gout |
| Arthritis | **Diuretic** | Hay fever |
| Assimilation | Dropsy | Insect bites, stings |
| Asthma | Elimination | **Kidney, congested** |
| **Bedwetting** | Eyes | **Kidney stones** |
| **Bladder** | Female problems | Laxative |
| Blood vessels | Fever | Liver, obstructions |
| Breath freshener | Flatulence-gas | Low blood pressure |
| Bruises | Fomentations | Menstruation, regulates |

| | | |
|---|---|---|
| Mucus, expels | **Prostate gland** | **Urination, painful** |
| Nervous system | Spleen | Venereal disease |
| Optic nerves | Syphilis | **Water retention** |
| Pain | Thyroid | Yellow jaundice |
| **Pituitary gland** | Tumors, prevent | |
| Poultice | **Urinary problems** | |

*Case History*

Whenever K. has a water retention problem, especially related to the menstrual cycle, she takes 2 capsules of parsley or an herbal diuretic combination that includes parsley. The problem is corrected within 30 minutes to an hour. She also has no problem with potassium depletion since parsley is high in potassium.

# PASSION FLOWER
## Antispasmodic, Nervine, Sedative

— acts as a mild sedative; relaxing.
— calming for high blood pressure.
— useful in nervousness, insomnia, headaches.
Has been used in the following:

| | | |
|---|---|---|
| **Alcoholism** | Heart | Menopause |
| Eye tension | **High blood pressure** | **Nerves** |
| Fever | Hysteria | Neuro-muscular |
| **Headache, nervous** | **Insomnia-sleep** | disorders |

# PEACH BARK
## Diuretic, Nervine.

— leaves are used for teas and poultices. Peach kernals are used for headaches.
— acts as a diuretic—relieves water retention.
— relieves inflammation in kidney and bladder complaints and used for other kidney and bladder problems.
— purifies the blood and cleanses toxins from the body.
— has calming effect on the nerves

Has been used for the following:

| | | |
|---|---|---|
| Abdominal inflammation | **Insomnia-sleep** | Stomach |
| Bladder | **Kidneys** | Uterus |
| Bronchitis | Laxative, mild | Whooping cough |
| Cholera | Morning sickness | Worms-parasites, expels |
| Colic | Nausea | |
| **Diuretic** | **Nerves** | Wounds |
| Fever | Poultice, leaves | Yellow jaundice |
| Flatulence-gas | Sores | |
| | Stomach ache | |

# PEPPERMINT
## Aromatic, Stimulant, Tonic.

Peppermint is a delicious mild tea. It is wonderful to use as a beverage—hot in the winter and cold in the summer. Dieters, it contains no calories.

— one of the oldest and most popular remedies for simple colic and minor bloat in children and adults.

— good for all digestive problems, helps stomach pain caused by indigestion and is soothing to the stomach.

— expels stomach and colon gas.

— excellent for fevers, flu, diarrhea, ulcers and colitis.

— strengthens nerves and heart muscles.

— cleanses and tones the body.

— can be used instead of aspirin for headaches.

— can take the place of coffee for a stimulant.

— promotes relaxation.

Has been used in the following:

| | | |
|---|---|---|
| Antispasmodic | Dizziness | Hysteria |
| **Bronchitis** | **Digestion** | **Nausea** |
| **Chills** | **Dysentery** | **Nerves,** soothes and strengthens |
| Cholera | **Fainting** | |
| **Colds** | **Fever** | **Stimulant** |
| **Colic** | **Flatulence-gas** | **Stomach** |
| **Colitis** | **Flu-influenza** | **Vomiting** |
| Countenance, pale | **Gastrointestinal** | Ulcers |
| **Diarrhea** | **Heart** | |
| | **Heart palpitations** | |

*Case History*

M.'s baby was suffering from a cold and a fever. She gave him peppermint tea in a bottle. Within a few minutes the baby was asleep and the fever had broken.

# POKE ROOT
## Alterative, Antibiotic, Depurant, Relaxant, Tonic.

— roots are used for medicinal purposes; the leaves are used for green drinks, salads, and poultices.

— powerful blood cleanser. Especially good in cleansing swollen infected glands.

— has persistent, flushing, cleansing action on the body which helps to expel waste and toxins. Tones the entire system.

— used to heal inflamed kidneys and relieve liver congestion.

— helps to break down mucus in intestines, sinus, and throughout the whole body.

— is an antibiotic, used in herbal antibiotic combinations.

— has an anti-cancer agent.

— has an appetite inhibiting agent.

— rich in many minerals, including iron.

Has been used in the following:

| | | |
|---|---|---|
| **Antibiotic** | **Glands, swollen** | **Mucus** |
| Biliousness | **or enlarged** | Poultice |
| Bony enlargements | Goiter | Scrofula |
| from injuries | Growth, abnormal | **Sinus** |
| **Blood cleanser** | **Infection** | Skin |
| **Breasts, caked** | Intestines | Spleen |
| Breasts, tumors | Itch, tea internally | Syphilis |
| Bronchitis | **Kidney, inflamed** | Thyroid |
| Cancer | Liniment | Weight loss |
| **Colds** | Liver | |
| **Eczema** | **Lymphatic System** | |

# PSYLLIUM

Psyllium has been called a "colon broom" because it scrubs the colon. It creates bulk and pulls putrefactive toxins from the sides of the intestines and colon. Drink plenty of water with it because it expands. Also take enemas or a good herbal laxative to help move the fecal matter and all of the psyllium out of the colon.

— acts as an intestinal lubricant.

— comes in bulk, stir in juice, or take capsules with plenty of water (at least 8 oz.)

Has been used in the following:

| | | |
|---|---|---|
| **Colitis** | Dysentery | **Intestinal tract** |
| **Colon cleanser** | Gonorrhea | **lubricant** |
| Constipation | Hemorrhage | Ulcers |
| Digestion | Hemorrhoids | Urinary |
| **Diverticulitis** | | |

# RED CLOVER
## Alterative, Blood Purifier, Sedative.

— relaxes nerves and the entire system. Can be used as a sedative.

— has been used to fight cancer. Found in herbal combinations used for cancer.

— wash for sores.

— good for a preventative of health problems.

— can be drunk freely.

Has been used in the following:

| | | |
|---|---|---|
| **Acne** | Leprosy | **Skin** |
| **Blood purifier** | Nerves | **Sores, wash** |
| **Boils** | Pellegra | Spasm |
| Bronchial | **Psoriasis** | Syphilis |
| **Cancer** | Rhuematism | Whooping Cough |
| Cough | Scarlet Fever | |

# REDMOND CLAY

Redmond Clay, a white clay, not an herb, is high in minerals and helps the body to utilize minerals and food. Red Clay is the most potent; green clay—second and white clay is more mild. It is better to start with white clay.

— relieves pain by pulling toxins from inflamed or toxic areas.

— reduces swelling. Used for external poultices called clay packs.

— clay packs have been used to reduce tumors in two to three days or sooner. Also reduces swollen liver. See Note.*

— clay packs—use small amounts of water until clay can be spread over the area. See Note.*

— used internally it detoxifies the body—especially the liver, cleanses the intestinal tract and expels worms.

— a daily dietary supplement of clay cleans the liver and the pancreas. Dissolve one teaspoon in glass of water overnight. Drink the next morning. (two to four capsules could be taken instead, but soaking the clay overnight activates the energy of clay.) This will take you back to the days of making mud pies, only this time you really get to eat them.

— good for any skin problem.

— always use with an herbal laxative.

*NOTE: When taking clay internally start with white clay. Also take clay internally for a couple of days before applying a clay pack. This is because clay sometimes pulls toxins to a head which forms a large sore and takes quite a long time to heal. If it is taken internally first, toxins start to be eliminated through the kidneys and colon.

Has been used in the following:

| | | |
|---|---|---|
| **Acne, pack** | Insect Bites, Stings | **Swelling,** pack |
| **Bee stings, pack** | **Intestinal tract,** | **Tumors** |
| **Boils** | **cleanses** | Varicose veins |
| **Burns** | Liver | Worms-parasites, |
| **Detoxification** | **Pain, pack** | expels |
| **Eczema** | **Poultice** | |
| Gastritis | **Skin** | |

*Case History*

During a painful kidney infection, Redmond Clay was mixed with mineral water and applied externally in the small part of the back over the kidneys. This was kept on overnight. By morning the pain was gone from the area. This was used each night until the kidney infection was completely gone. Kidney and infection fighting herbs were taken internally during this time.

Redmond Clay mixed with water was put on a grease burn on the face and the pain left instantly.

# RED RASPBERRY
## Alterative, Astringent, Stomachic, Tonic.

Red Raspberry is used as a basic herbal foundation for all female organs and problems. It is in many female combinations.

— strengthens wall of uterus and entire female reproductive system.

— decreases profuse menstrual flow.

— good during all months of pregnancy. Alleviates morning sickness and nausea (see remedies Pregnancy Chapter). Has been used as a preventative for hemorrhaging during labor. Assists labor, makes delivery easier and relieves afterpains. Tones and regulates before, during and after childbirth.

— increases and enriches milk for lactation, can be combined with Marshmallow tea.

— Raspberry tea is mild and pleasant to taste. It is good for stomach aches and bowel problems in children. For diarrhea in babies.

— soothing to stomach and bowels and cankerous conditions of mucous membranes in the alimentary canal.

— high mineral and vitamin source.

Has been used in the following:

| | | |
|---|---|---|
| **Afterpains, childbirth** | Diabetes | **Flu-influenza** |
| **Antacid** | **Diarrhea** | **Gastritis** |
| Bronchitis | **Digestion** | Hemorrhoids |
| Cankers | Douche | **Labor pains** |
| **Childbirth** | Dysentary | Leucorrhea |
| Cholera | Eyewash | Measles |
| **Colds** | **Female problems** | **Menstrual flow,** |
| Constipation | **Fevers** | **decreases** |
| **Coughs** | **Flatulence-Gas** | **Miscarriage** |

| Mouth sores | **Pregnancy** | **Uterus, strengthens** |
|---|---|---|
| **Mucous membranes** | Stomach ache | **& tones** |
| **Nausea** | Throat, sore | Vaginal discharge |
| Nerves | Ulcers | |
| **Nursing** | Urinary problems | |

### *Case History*

L. was terribly nauseous during the first months of pregnancy. She felt weak and was receiving B-12 shots from her doctor. She started drinking 3 to 4 cups of Red Raspberry tea every day, the nausea went away. She was able to start eating again and felt the tea helped her during delivery too.

## ROSEHIPS
### Aperient, Astringent, Stomachic.

— good for stress.
— much vitamin C, contains vitamin C complex (see Vit. C)
— infection fighter.
Has been used in the following:

| **Arteriosclerosis** | Contagious diseases | Insect bites, stings |
|---|---|---|
| Arthritis | Emphysema | Kidneys |
| Bruises | **Fever** | **Stress** |
| Circulation | Heart | Yellow jaundice |
| **Colds** | **Infections** | |

## ROSEMARY
### Antispasmodic, Astringent, Emmenagogue, · Stimulant, Tonic.

— used in shampoos to help prevent baldness. The oil is used as perfume for ointments.
— long used remedy for colds, coughs and nervous conditions especially nervous headaches.
— wash for mouth, gums, and sore throat.

— used for female problems.
— used for high blood pressure.
Has been used in the following:

| | | |
|---|---|---|
| Baldness | **Headaches, nervous** | Shampoo |
| **Colds** | High blood pressure | Throat, sore |
| Coughs | Miscarriage | Weight loss |
| Female problems | Nervous conditions | |
| Gums | Nightmares | |

# SAFFLOWERS
## Diaphoretic, Digestant, Laxative.

Safflower is a natural digestive aid. It aids in the utilization of sugar in fruits and also utilization of oils. It contains natural hydrochloric acid.

— soothes and coats the entire digestive tract.
— helps heal the walls of the intestines in diverticulitis.
— stimulates glandular secretions in intestines.
— relieves gas.
— has mild laxative action in bowels
— acts as diuretic
— has ability to remove sticky phlegm from body.
— helps heal lesions
— helps cholesterol levels in body.
— neutralizes uric acid and lactic acid. Uric acid holds hardened deposits in joints that lead to gout and arthritis. These acids also are a cause of kidney stones.
— **Safflowers and Saffron can be used inter-changeably.**
Has been used in the following:

| | | |
|---|---|---|
| **Acid Stomach** | Flu-Influenza | Menstruation, |
| Appetite | Flatulence-Gas | tardy |
| **Arthritis** | **Gout** | Perspiration, |
| Colds | Heartburn | promotes |
| Diabetes | **Hypoglycemia** | Scarlet Fever |
| **Digestion** | **Kidney Stones** | Skin Disease |
| Diuretic | **Lesions** | Water Retention |
| Diverticulitis | Liver | Yellow Jaundice |
| Fevers | Measles | |

# SAGE
## Alterative, Diuretic, Tonic.

There are two kinds of sage - garden and wild.

**Garden Sage:**

— used to cook with, good for digestion.

— the tea has been used as a hair rinse to return hair to its natural color and for baldness.

— used for nerve related problems such as headaches.

**Wild or Wood Sage:**

— used mostly for medicinal reasons. Also used as a tonic.

— high in minerals.

— good for nerves.

— stops profuse or irregular menstrual flow when combined with yarrow (see Women Only Chapter.)

— good for circulation and the heart.

— used for poultices for tumors.

— the tea is used for a gargle for sore or ulcerated throats, as a wash for wounds, for fevers, coughs, colds and pneumonia.

— if you gather it from the country side, be sure to get it away from highways where it won't be contaminated by exhaust fumes.

Has been used in the following:

| | | |
|---|---|---|
| **Bladder** | **Heart** | Pneumonia |
| Bronchitis | Hoarseness | Skin |
| Circulation | Impotency | **Sores, cleans** |
| Colds | Insect bites, stings | **and heals** |
| Coughs | **Kidneys** | Stomach |
| Dandruff | Laryngitis | Throat, sore |
| Depression | Liver | Tonsillitis |
| Diarrhea | Lungs | Ulcers |
| **Digestion** | Menstruation, | Worms-parasites, |
| Dyspepsia | profuse, regulates | expels |
| Fevers | Mouth sores | Wounds, bleeding |
| Flatulence-gas | Nausea | Yeast Infections |
| Flu-influenza | Nerves | |
| Gargle | Night sweats | |
| **Hair tonic** | Nursing, to stop | |
| Headache | Perspiration, | |
| | promotes | |

# SARSAPARILLA
## Alterative, Diuretic, Hormonal, Relaxant, Stimulant, Tonic.

— excellent in balancing hormones in both males and females. Contains the male hormones testosterone (an important hair growing hormone), progesterone, and cortin; stimulates the action of estrogen in females.
— has been used in rheumatism and gout.
— increases flow of urine.
— used in blood purifier combinations.
— promotes perspiration when taken hot.
Has been used in the following:

| | | |
|---|---|---|
| Age spots | Eyewash | Inflammation, |
| Aging | Fever | internal |
| **Blood purifier** | Flatulence-gas | Perspiration |
| Boils | Gout | Psoriasis |
| Catarrh | **Hair growth** | Rheumatism |
| Cleansing | Heartburn | Ringworm |
| Colds | **Hormones, balance** | Skin |
| **Diuretic** | Impotency | Venereal diseases |

# SAW PALMETTO
## Antiseptic, Cardiac, Hormonal, Sedative, Tonic.

— hormone herb; has a good effect on all diseases of the reproductive organs in both males and females; has been known to enlarge underdeveloped breasts in some women.
— benefits all glandular tissue.
— helps to rid body of excess mucus from head, sinus, and lungs.
Has been used in the following:

| | | |
|---|---|---|
| Alcoholism | Flu-influenza | **Reproductive** |
| Arthritis | **Glandular tissue** | **organs** |
| Asthma | **Hormones, regulates** | Throat, sore |
| Bright's disease | Mucus | Weight, gain |
| Bronchitis | Nerves | Whooping cough |
| Colds | | |
| Diabetes | | |

# SCULLCAP
## Antispasmodic, Diuretic, Nervine, Sedative, Tonic.

— one of the best nerve herbs; has a calming effect especially for worry and emotional disturbances. It has a tonic influence which tones and soothes the entire nervous system.

— brings on a natural sleep.

— aids in cases of spasms, tremors, twitching of muscles, epilepsy and convulsions.

— good for digestion and circulation.

— should be taken for long periods of time to overcome any of the above problems. Has no harmful side effects.

— has a diuretic property which draws out uric acid. This helps the nervous system in rheumatism, gout, or neuritis.

Has been used in the following:

| | | |
|---|---|---|
| **Alcoholism** | Hypoglycemia | Rabies |
| **Circulation** | Hysteria | Relaxant |
| Convulsions | Insect bites, stings | **Rheumatism** |
| **Digestion** | Mental illness | Sexual desire, undue |
| **Diuretic** | Mumps | **Insomnia-sleep** |
| Epilepsy | **Muscles twitch** | Smoking |
| Fits | **Nerves** | Snake bites |
| **Gout** | **Neuritis** | Spasms |
| **Hangover** | Pain | Stress |
| Headache | Palsy | Thyroid |
| Heart strengthener | Paralysis | Tremors |
| Hypersensitivity | | |

# SLIPPERY ELM
## Demulcent, Diuretic, Emollient, Nutritive, Tonic.

Slippery elm is an amazing, mild-flavored, highly nutritious herb. It is used in many combinations and poultices not only because of its medicinal properties but also because of its cohesive quality that helps hold the other herbs together. The dried inner bark is the part used.

— in case of a famine, it would be an excellent herb to store and to forage for eating.

— mucilaginous and expands when mixed with water. Does not mix easily, use a blender, wire whip, fork, or shake in bottle, etc.

— should be taken with lots of water.

— contact healer both internally and externally. Coats relaxes, and heals all inflamed tissues including irritated and inflamed mucous membranes of stomach, bowels, and kidney.

— a gentle herb—one of the best for diarrhea especially for babies. It normalizes the stools, soothes, coats, and heals the entire intestinal tract lining.

— used in enemas for scalding diarrhea because of soothing and healing qualities. (see remedies Baby Chapter.) The flavor hints of burnt caramel candy—most babies willingly eat a Slippery Elm mixture.

— good for ulcers and delicate stomachs

— great for hiatal hernias. Must be taken in tea form or powder stirred in water for this. Capsules would dissolve in the stomach and the hernia would not be coated since it is above the stomach.

— used for vaginal douches. (see Women Only Chapter)

Has been used in the following:

| | | |
|---|---|---|
| Adrenal glands | Eczema | Pneumonia |
| Asthma | Esophagus, sore | Poultices |
| Bladder | Eyes | Poison Ivy, external |
| Boils | Fever | Rashes |
| **Bowels** | Flatulence-gas | Respiratory system |
| Bronchitis | Flu-influenza | Sex stimulant |
| Burns | **Food** | **Sores** |
| Cancer | Gangrene | Stomach acidity |
| **Colitis** | **Gastrointestinal** | **Throat, sore** |
| **Colon** | Hay fever | **Tonsillitis** |
| **Constipation** | Hemorrhage | Tumors |
| Cough | **Hemorrhoids** | **Ulcers** |
| Cramps | Herpes | Urinary tract |
| Cystitis | **Hiatal hernia** | Vaginal discharge |
| Demulcent | Hoarseness | Vaginal douche |
| Diabetes | Inflammation | Venereal disease |
| **Diaper rash** | Intestines | Whooping cough |
| **Diarrhea** | Kidneys | Worms-parasites, expels |
| **Digestion** | Lungs, pain | Wounds |
| Diphtheria | Mucous membranes | Yellow Jaundice |
| **Diverticulitis** | Mucus, removes | |
| **Dysentery** | Nutrition | |

*Case History*

G. had internal hemorrhoids that were sore and bleeding. She mixed a small retention enema of Slippery Elm. (see Hemorrhoids, Ailments.) The bleeding and pain stopped within minutes.

Herbs are also used with animals. When lambs are born they have a tendency to get diarrhea (scours). Many times the lambs die. S. fed her lambs Slippery Elm mixture (See diarrhea Baby chapter). The diarrhea was corrected very quickly.

# TAHEEBO (PAU D'ARCO)
## Alterative, Antibiotic, Depurative, Tonic, Viricide.

Taheebo comes from the inner bark of the Red Lapacho tree in the Andes of South America. It has been used for centuries. Theodoro Meyer of the National University of Tucuman, Argentina was the first modern scientist to study Taheebo's chemical composition. He found it contained XYLOIDIN-an antibiotic with viricidal properties. Also contains LAPACHOL-an element noted for its anti-tumor activity.

— used for many disorders, considered an "everything" herb.

— make tea of 1 heaping Tb. steeped for 5-20 minutes in 4-6 cups of water and drink.

— there is some evidence that some cancers are caused by virus. Many people use Taheebo in fighting cancer.

— used for all skin diseases.

— good for sores, even old ones, used externally.

Has been used in the following:

| | | |
|---|---|---|
| Anemia | Diabetes | Kidneys |
| Asthma | Dizziness | Leukemia |
| Arteriosclerosis | **Eczema** | Liver |
| Baldness | Gastritis | Malaria |
| Blood builder | Gonorrhea | Osteomyelitis |
| **Blood purifier** | Hemorrhages | Pain |
| Bronchitis | Hemorrhoids | Parkinson's disease |
| **Cancer, all types** | **Herpes** | Polyps, intestinal |
| Circulation | Hernias | **Prostate** |
| Colitis | Indigestion | Psoriasis |
| Colon | Inflammation | Rheumatism |
| Cystitis | Impotency | Ring worm |

| Scabies | Syphilis | Ulcers |
|---|---|---|
| Skin | **Tonic** | Ulceration of |
| Sores | Tumors | intestines |
| Spleen | Typhoid Fever | Wounds |

# THYME
## Antiseptic, Nervine, Tonic.

— Thyme can be used to season food. It is good in Italian dishes, in soups, stocks, meats and vegetables. Adding thyme to your food gives more nutrition, some beneficial medicinal properties, as well as flavor.

— removes mucus from head, lungs, and respiratory passages.

— has a soothing, sedative action on nerves.

— fights infection and is anti-fungus.

— expels worms.

— used in breaking alcoholic habit.

— tonic for stomach.

— pain-reliever for migraine headaches when combined with Fenugreek.

Has been used in the following:

| | | |
|---|---|---|
| **Alcoholic** | Gastrointestinal | **Respiratory** |
| Anemia | Gout | Rheumatism |
| Asthma | **Hangover, migraine** | Sinus |
| Athlete's foot | **Headache** | **Stomach** |
| Bowel | Heartburn | **Stomach cramps** |
| Bronchitis | **Infection** | Tumors |
| Bruises | Insomnia | Uterus |
| Colic | Lungs | Warts |
| Cramps | Menstruation, | Whooping cough |
| Diarrhea | painful | **Worms-parasites,** |
| Digestion | **Mucus, removes** | **expels** |
| Fever | Nerves | Wounds, stab |
| Gastritis | Odors | |

# TURKEY RHUBARB
## Astringent, Cathartic.

— also called Rhubarb Root, but don't confuse it with the domestic Rhubarb plant.
— cleanses alimentary canal and entire digestive tract.
— improves digestion and appetite.
— stimulates peristaltic action and glandular secretions.
— good for relaxing colon, for pain, and relaxing bowels in appendicitis.
— purgative to intestinal tract. Has been used in enemas and taken by mouth to help move blockages in the colon.
Has been used in the following:

| | | |
|---|---|---|
| Alimentary canal | Diarrhea | **Laxative** |
| Appendicitis | **Digestion** | **Purgative** |
| Appetite | **Duodenum** | Stomach, tonic |
| **Colon** | **Hemorrhoids** | |
| Colon Blockage | **Intestines** | |

# UVA URSI
## Antiseptic, Astringent, Diuretic, Tonic.

— effective in all kidney disorders, including mucus discharges with pus and blood.
— stimulates kidneys. Strengthens and tones mucous membranes or urinary passages.
— solvent for kidney stones.
— has healing action on genito-urinary organs.
— cleanses and strengthens the spleen.
— a disgestive stimulant.
— good for female problems.
Has been used in the following:

| | | |
|---|---|---|
| **Bedwetting** | Dysentery | Lumbago |
| **Bladder** | Female problems | Menstruation, |
| Bright's disease | Gonorrhea | profuse |
| Bronchitis | Hemorrhoids | Mucous membranes |
| Cystitis | **Kidney** | Nephritis |
| Diabetes | **Kidney stones** | Pancreas |
| **Digestion** | Liver | Prostate gland |

| Spleen | Urinary organs | Venereal disease |
|--------|----------------|------------------|
| Syphilis | Vaginal discharge | Weight loss |

# VALERIAN ROOT
## Antispasmodic, Diuretic, Nervine, Stimulant, Tonic

Valerian Root is a powerful, effective antispasmodic. It quiets, calms, and has a healing effect on the nervous system. Valerian Root is a marvelous weapon against stress and nerves.

— promotes sleep if taken at night. Has no narcotic effect.

— relieves pain.

— good to normalize heart palpitations, slows action of heart while strengthening it. Good for circulatory system.

— stimulates secretion and peristaltic action of stomach and intestines.

— antiflatulent (gas) for adults and infants.

— used for children with measles and scarlet fever for restlessness and pain.

Has been used in the following:

| | | |
|---|---|---|
| Acne | Coughs | **Insomnia-sleep** |
| **Afterpains, childbirth** | **Cramps, menstrual** | Intestines |
| **Alcoholism** | Digestion | Measles |
| **Antispasmodic** | Drug addiction | Menstruation |
| **Arthritis, pain** | Epilepsy | brings on suppressed |
| **Bladder** | Fevers | when taken hot. |
| Blood pressure | Flatulence-gas | **Muscle Spasms, pain** |
| Bronchitis | Hangover | **Nervine** |
| Childhood diseases | **Headaches** | **Nervous debility** |
| Circulatory system | Head congestion | **Pain** |
| **Colic** | Heart burn | Palsy |
| **Colds** | **Heart palpitations** | Paralysis |
| **Contagious diseases** | Hypochondriac | **Restlessness** |
| Convulsions | Hysteria | Scarlet fever |

Shock                          Ulcers
Stomach, ulcerated             Worms-parasites,
                                   expels

# WHITE OAK BARK
## Antiseptic, Astringent, Diuretic, Tonic.

— used in tea form as an antiseptic to disinfect wounds, sores, and scabs to prevent infection and kill germs.

— used in douches for leucorrhea and other vaginal discharges and in enemas for hemorrhoids. It is especially effective for bleeding hemorrhoids. (see ailments.)

— used with Goldenseal as a mouth rinse for oral surgery. (see ailments)

— good for internal and external tumors and swellings.

— reduces varicose veins—take internally and use fomentations externally. (see ailments.)

— normalizes liver, kidneys and spleen. Increases flow of urine. Removes kidney stones and gall stones. Helps with all kidney problems including blood in the urine and bladder infections.

— for goiter use fomentation and take internally.

— stops hemorrhages in lungs, stomach, bowels, and spitting up of blood.

— curbs excessive menstrual flow.

— brings fevers down.

— will expel pin worms.

Has been used in the following:

| | | |
|---|---|---|
| **Bladder infections** | **Gall stones** | Nausea |
| **Bladder, ulcerated** | Glandular swellings | **Oral surgery** |
| **Bleeding** | Goiter | Pinworms |
| Bowels, bleeding | Hemorrhages | **Pyorrhea** |
| Bruises | Hemorrhoids | Rectum |
| Cancer, prostate | Insect bites, stings | **Skin** |
| **Diuretic** | **Kidney stones** | **Sores** |
| Diarrhea | Leucorrhea | Snake bites |
| **Douches** | **Liver** | Spleen |
| **Enemas** | Lungs | Stomach |
| Fever blisters | Menstrual flow, | Teeth, loose |
| Fevers | profuse | Thrush |
| Gall Bladder | **Mouth sores** | Tonsilitis |

| | | |
|---|---|---|
| Toothache | **Urine, bloody** | Wounds |
| Tumors | Uterus | Vaginal discharge |
| Ulcers | **Varicose veins** | Yeast infection |
| **Urinary problems** | Venereal disease | Yellow Jaundice |

## *Case History:*

F. had such bad varicose veins she couldn't even get out of bed. She took 8 capsules of White Oak Bark a day. There was a dramatic change in her varicose veins. She now takes 8 a day regularly.

## WHITE WILLOW
### Analgesic, Anti-inflammatory, Antipyretic, Astringent.

In 1827, Leroux, a French Chemist extracted a substance he called "Salicin" from the bark of the White Willow tree. Salicin is the pain relieving, main active ingredient of White Willow. In Germany, 1890, Felix Hofman and Fredrick Bayer used White Willow and found a related compound to Salicin-Acetyl-Salicylic Acid. In 1899, this product, eventually called aspirin (Bayers Aspirin), was marketed commercially when Bayer and Hofman switched to synthetic sources, using phenol and sodium hydroxide, instead of the natural willow.

Aspirin, the most used drug in the world, is simply a synthetic form of White Willow. Some side effects of aspirin are interference of blood clotting processes, stomach upset, stomach bleeding, ulcers, hives, asthma, hearing loss, dizziness, shortness of breath, anemia, pregnancy problems, urinary infections, and Reyes Syndrome.

Salicin or White Willow is natural and is converted by the body to Salicylic Acid, which is mild to the stomach. Salicylic Acid performs the same role in the body as aspirin, but doesn't have the side effects of aspirin.

The Indians have been using Willow for centuries. It is mentioned in Egyptian Papyri, and Hippocrates prescribed it for pain and fever, etc . . . The historical uses of White Willow Bark are extensive.

— contains other organic compounds not found in aspirin which helps the body use Salicin with no apparent harmful side effects.

**Three Major Uses of White Willow Bark**

1. Reduces fever
2. Pain reliever
3. Anti-inflammatory (used for rheumatism and arthritis)

Has been used in the following:

| | | |
|---|---|---|
| **Anti-inflammatory** | Eye, inflamed | Malaria |
| **Arthritis** | and infected | **Muscles, sore** |
| Asthma | **Fevers** | **Nerves** |
| Astringent | **Flu-influenza** | Nosebleed |
| Chills | **Gout** | Ovarian pain |
| **Colds** | Hayfever | **Pain** |
| Corns | **Headache** | **Rheumatism** |
| Dandruff | Heartburn | **Tonsillitis** |
| **Earaches** | Infection | Worms-parasites, |
| Eczema | Inflammation | Wounds |

# WOOD BETONY
## Alterative, Antirheumatic, Astringent, Nervine, Tonic.

— good for all head and face pain including headaches. (For migraine headaches see Fenugreek and Thyme)
— good for all nerve problems. Relaxes muscles and nerves in the back of the head and neck.
— good for heartburn and indigestion.
— opens obstructions of liver and spleen.
— mildly stimulating to heart.
— cleans impurities from blood.
— expels worms.

Has been used in the following:

| | | |
|---|---|---|
| Asthma | Dropsy | Indigestion |
| Bladder | Epilepsy | Insanity |
| Colds | Fainting | Insect bites, stings |
| Colic | Flu-influenza | Liver |
| Consumption | Gout | Lungs |
| Convulsion | Headache | **Nerves** |
| Delirium | Heart | Neuralgia |
| Diarrhea | Heartburn | **Pain** |

| Palsy | Varicose veins | Yellow Jaundice |
| Rheumatism | Worms-parasites, | |
| Spleen | expels | |

# YARROW
## Astringent, Diaphoretic, Diuretic, Stimulant, Tonic.

Yarrow is an important herb to have in storage in your home. The comment was made that it would be one of the only things that works against the coming plagues,which would be flu type diseases. Yarrow is unsurpassed for flu and fevers.

— used abundantly at the beginning of a cold it will usually break it up within 24 hours.

— especially good for fevers-produces perspiration. Opens pores and has relaxing action on skin.

— for fever must be drunk warm or take capsules with warm water or peppermint tea. Yarrow tea is bitter to the taste, but effective.

— good for all childhood diseases. A yarrow ointment or tea is used for sores, including chicken pox and smallpox, also old wounds.

— healing to glaundular system. Regulates and tones liver.

— relieves kidneys problems, infections and mucus discharge from bladder.

— equalizes circulation.

— used in fomentations for external hemorrhoids or inject one ounce of the tea in a retention enema for internal hemorrhoids. (see Hemorrhoids)

— corrects diarrhea in infants.

— healing and soothing to all mucous membranes.

— benefits respiratory problems, including bleeding from lungs.

— combined with sage, it is good for profuse or irregular menstruation. (see For Women Only.)

Has been used in the following:

| Arthritis | Bright's disease | Cancer |
| Bladder | Bronchitis | Catarrh |
| Blood purifier | Burns | **Chicken pox** |
| Bowels | Bursitis | **Colds** |

Colon

Congestion

Contagious diseases

Diabetes

Diarrhea

Douche

Dysentery

Dyspepsia

Ear infections

Enemas

**Female problems**

**Fever**

Flatulence-gas

**Flu-influenza**

Hair loss

Hemorrhage

Hemorrhoids

Kidneys

Leucorrhea

Liver

Lungs, bleeding

Measles

**Menstruation,
     profuse, irregular**

**Mucous membrane**

**Pleurisy**

**Pneumonia**

Smallpox

Spleen

Throat, sore

Typhoid

Ulcers

Uterus

**Urinary problems**

**Urine, suppressed**

Vaginal discharge

Wounds

Yellow Jaundice

# YELLOW DOCK
## Alterative, Astringent, Laxative, Tonic.

— blood cleanser, purifier, and builder; tones the entire system.

— high in Vitamin C and iron compounds-one of the best blood builders.

— good for all skin problems.

— dissolves mucus and moves it through kidneys.

— excellent cleanser of lymphatic system.

— dissolves glandular and other tumors. Kills parasites which contribute to cancer.

— used for hepatitis. (see ailments.)

— the plant is edible. The leaves are used for green drink and other eating.

Has been used in the following:

Acne

**Anemia**

Arsenic poisoning

Bladder

Bleeding

Blood purifier
   and builder

Boils

Bowels, bleeding

Bronchitis

Cancer

Catarrh

Chicken Pox

**Cough**

Diarrhea

Ears, infected

Endurance

Energy

Eyelids, ulcerated

Fevers

Gall bladder

Hemorrhage

**Hepatitis**

Itching

Laryngitis

Leukemia

Leprosy

**Liver congestion**

Lungs

**Lymphatic system**

Mental fatigue

**Mucus, expels**

**Pituitary**

Poison Ivy, Oak

Psoriasis

Scarlet fever

Scurvy

**Skin**

**Sores**

Spleen

Stomach, sour

Swellings

Syphilis

Thyroid

Tumors

Ulcers

Venereal disease

Vitality

**Worms-parasites,**
  expels.

**Yellow Jaundice**

# CHAPTER 2

# *Herbal Combinations*

## TINCTURES

Tinctures are herbs aged in alcohol or apple cider vinegar. They are more concentrated and easily assimilated in this liquid form. (See Herbal Preparations)

### Single Herbs in Tincture Form

Some single herbs in tincture form are: Black Walnut, Capsicum, Hawthorne Berries, Licorice Root, Lobelia, Royal Jelly/Dong Quai, Siberian Ginseng.

## COMBINATIONS OF HERBS IN TINCTURE FORM

### Anti-Spasmodic and Nerve Combinations

1. _____ Valerian Root, Aniseed, Lobelia, Brigham Tea, Black Walnut Hulls, Licorice, Ginger.
   — highly concentrated, works very quickly. A few drops to ¼-½ teaspoon every two hours has been used for adults.
   — helps feed the nerves and gives a calm feeling. Described by one person as "just taking a burden off your shoulders."
MOST COMMON USES

| | | |
|---|---|---|
| Anti-spasmodic | Coughing | Spastic Conditions |
| Arthritis | Insomnia-Sleep | Stress |
| Convulsions | Nerves | |

2. _____ Chickweed, Black Cohosh, Goldenseal, Lobelia, Scullcap, Brigham Tea, Licorice.
— used for ear drops to relieve ear ache and fight infection.
— used for nerves, antispasmodic.
MOST COMMON USES
Antispasmodic          Equilibrium          Nerves
Ear problems

# HERBAL COMBINATIONS

### Allergy Combinations

1. _____ Blessed Thistle, Black Cohosh, Scullcap, Pleurisy Root.

2. _____ Brigham Tea, Marshmallow, Goldenseal, Chaparral, Burdock, Parsley, Cayenne, Lobelia.
— these combinations stimulate natural antihistamines, also act as natural antihistamines in the body and cleanse the affected areas.
— works well with Mega Vitamin A, C and Pantothenic Acid, which act as natural antihistamines.
— has been known to help some acne problems.
MOST COMMON USES
Allergies          Hay Fever          Sinus
Asthma          Mucus          Sinus Headaches

### Case History:

J. had had chronic allergy and sinus problems for years. He also needed to have allergy shots yearly for the problem. He used antihistamines and sprays constantly. After using the Allergy Combination #1, his head began to drain, then clear. It was the first time in years he had had any effective relief.

### Arthritis Combinations

1. _____ Bromelain Powder, Yucca, Comfrey, Alfalfa, Black Cohosh, Yarrow, Capsicum, Chaparral, Lobelia, Burdock, Century Herb.

2. _____ Hydrangea, Brigham Tea, Chaparral, Lobelia, Burdock, Sarsparilla, Wild Lettuce, Valerian,

Wormwood, Black Cohosh, Capsicum, Black Walnut, Yucca, Scullcap.

— often relieves the pain and stiffness of arthritis and helps to remove the congestion that causes the arthritis.

— arthritis is a chronic condition. Best results are achieved using arthritis combinations with compatible vitamins, minerals and diet. (See Ailments)

— comes in regular or concentrated capsules.

MOST COMMON USES

| | | |
|---|---|---|
| Arthritis | Gout | Rheumatism |
| Bursitis | | |

### *Case History:*

K.'s 90 year old father was in much pain with arthritis and was confined to a wheel chair. He started taking arthritis combination #1 and noticed less pain within six weeks. He was able to get out of his wheelchair and walk with a walker and finally a cane.

### Blood Builder Combinations

1. _____ Kelp, Alfalfa, Dandelion.

2. _____ Yellow Dock, Red Beet, Nettle, Mullein, Strawberry Leaves, Lobelia.

— Yellow Dock is high in iron. Dandelion contains the nutritive salts in the blood which balances the blood. These combinations build the blood.

— used by pregnant women for anemia.

— #1 used to improve hair, skin and nails.

MOST COMMON USES

| | | |
|---|---|---|
| Anemia | Glandular balance | Minerals |
| Endurance | Liver | Pregnancy |
| Energy | | |

### *Case History:*

J. had always suffered with anemia during her pregnancies. The next pregnancy she took Blood Builder Combination #2 and had no problem with anemia. She has felt better, had more energy and slept better.

## Blood Pressure and Heart Combinations

1. _____ Capsicum, Garlic.

2. _____ Hawthorne, Garlic, Cayenne.

3. _____ Capsicum, Parsley, Ginger, Ginseng, Goldenseal.

— These herbs help to strengthen blood vessels and equalize blood pressure.

— Helps dissolve plaque in arterial walls.

— Aids veins to regain elasticity.

— The cayenne (capsicum) has an immediate beneficial effect on the heart and then strengthens the rest of the circulatory system. (See also Hawthorne)

MOST COMMON USES

| | | |
|---|---|---|
| Blood pressure, equalizer | Flu, combinations #1 and #2 | Heart High blood pressure |
| Energy | General tonic | |

*Case History:*

L. had high blood pressure. She started taking 2 capsules three times a day of combination #1. She has had no more high blood pressure problems since then. She was able to get off her blood pressure prescription medicine.

## Blood Purifier Combinations

1. _____ Yellow Dock, Dandelion, Burdock, Licorice, Chaparral, Red Clover, Barberry, Cascara Sagrada, Yarrow, Sarsaparilla

2. _____ Red Clover, Chaparral, Licorice, Poke Root, Peach Bark, Oregon Grape, Stillingia, Cascara Sagrada.

— helps to carry toxins away from the cells to the eliminating organs and nutrients to the cells.

— helps cleanse the blood to maintain health.

MOST COMMON USES

| | | |
|---|---|---|
| Acne | Chronic Problems | Poison Ivy, Oak |
| Anemia | Contagious Diseases | Respiratory System |
| Blood Purifier | Endocrine System | Ringworm |
| Boils | Gangrene | Skin |
| Cancer | Liver | Tumors |

*Case History:*

H. had chronic acne. He started taking Blood Purifier Combination #1. At first the acne seemed to get worse. After 3 or 4 weeks it began to clear up. He also took enemas and went on a short (5 day) juice fast during this time to help clear the toxins out of his system. (See also Acne, Ailments Chapter)

## Calcium Combinations

1. _____ Comfrey, Alfalfa, Oatstraw, Irish Moss, Horsetail, Lobelia.

2. _____ Horsetail, Comfrey, Oat Straw, Lobelia.

3. _____ White Oak Bark, Comfrey, Mullein, Black Walnut, Marshmallow, Queen of the Meadow, Wormwood, Lobelia, Scullcap.

— high in calcium and other elements that help calcium be assimilated.

— #3 is also used for poultices (See poultice combinations)

MOST COMMON USES

| | | |
|---|---|---|
| Arthritis | Cramps | Menstruation |
| Bed Wetting | Eczema | Muscle Spasms |
| Bone Knitter | Fingernails | Pain |
| Broken Bones | Gout | Pregnancy |
| Bursitis | Insomnia-sleep | Rheumatism |
| Cartilage | Lactation | Teeth |

*Case History:*

— A small girl complained to her mother often about her legs hurting. The little girls legs hurt so much that she cried. Her mother tried Calcium Combination #1 and within hours the child's legs had stopped hurting and she was feeling much better. With Calcium you see quick results. The mother continues to give the child this combination for these growing pains.

— A 78 year old man was having problems with painful charley horses. He had been trying many different kinds of Calcium supplements without alleviating the problem. He tried Calcium Combination #1 and the charley horses went away. Note: If your body cannot assimilate the supplements you are using they will do you no good.

### Colitis Combination

1. _____ Marshmallow, Slippery Elm, Comfrey, Lobelia, Ginger, Wild Yam.
   — very calming, soothing and healing to the intestinal tract, stops pain, and coats intestinal lining. (See also Ulcer Combination)
   — helps to normalize bowel action.

MOST COMMON USES

Colitis                    Ulcers


### Digestion Combinations

1. _____ Papaya Fruit, Peppermint Leaves.

2. _____ Hydrochloric Acid, Betaine, Pepsin.

3. _____ Pepsin, Pancreatin, Mycozyme, Papain, Bromelain, Bile Salt, Lipase, Betaine, HCL.

4. _____ Fennel, Wild Yam, Peppermint, Ginger, Papaya, Catnip, Spearmint, Lobelia.

5. _____ Comfrey, Pepsin. (See Intestinal Cleanser)
   — good for all digestive disorders and for diseases where people need maximum nutrition. Most people suffering from chronic problems also have poor digestion.
   — after about age 35 our enzyme activity starts to slow down.
   — enzymes and digestive herbs help prevent cancer.
   — used as an anti-gas formula, and for heartburn. The synthetic antacid tablets available in the drugstore are alkalis used to neutralize stomach acid. When the acid is neutralized the food in the stomach is not digested and then "sits" on the stomach. People who continually use antacid tablets create a self-perpetuating monster of acid, antacid; more acid, more antacid, etc . . . It's better to aid the stomach in digestion rather than just neutralizing acid.

MOST COMMON USES

Cancer Preventative      Flatulence-Gas         Heartburn
Digestion


### *Case History:*

L. had heartburn, gas and indigestion until she took 1 or 2 tablets of Digestion Combination #3 with each meal.

**Energy and Fitness Combination**

1. _____ Siberian Ginseng, Ho Shou Wu, Black Walnut, Licorice Root, Genetian Root, Comfrey, Fennel, Bee Pollen, Bayberry, Myrrh Gum, Peppermint, Safflower Flowers, Eucalyptus, leaves, Lemon Grass, Capsicum Fruit.
   — energy and endurance, builds and strengthens body, increases work capacity.
   — used as an athletic formula for better performance.
MOST COMMON USES

| | | |
|---|---|---|
| Athletic Builder | Endurance | Pick-me-up |
| Energy | | |

**Energy and Memory Combinations**

1. _____ Capsicum, Ginseng, Gota Kola.

2. _____ Blessed Thistle, Periwinkle, Blue Vervain, Lobelia, Ginger, Capsicum.
   —stimulates circulation to the brain.
   — gives energy and endurance.
   — prevents and alleviates senility.
   — energy and memory combination #1 has been used while studying and before tests for better mental alertness.
MOST COMMON USES

| | | |
|---|---|---|
| Energy | Longevity | Pick-me-up |
| Endurance | Memory | Senility |

*Case History:*

J. was having times when she could not remember who she was or where she was. This problem went away when she took Energy and Memory #1. She has not had this problem for years. She continues to take the combination.

**Eyewash Combinations**

1. _____ Goldenseal, Bayberry, Eyebright.

2. _____ Goldenseal, Bayberry, Eyebright, Red Raspberry, Capsicum.
   — used as an eyewash. Steep as a tea, strain and cool before using. (See Eyes in Ailments)

— soothing to tired eyes.

NOTE:   Sometimes this washing will draw impurities from the eyes so that the eyesight seems filmy after using and matter will come out. After toxins and unwanted mucus clear up the eyesight will become clear.

— it is possible that some cataracts are caused by mucus hardening over the cornea.

— also used internally to fight eye infections and improve eyesight.

MOST COMMON USES

| | | |
|---|---|---|
| Cataracts | Glaucoma | Vision aid |
| Eye infections | | |

### *Case History:*

A new born baby had a closed tear duct. Eyewash Combination #1 was made into a tea, strained, cooled and dropped into the baby's eye with an eye dropper or piece of sterile cotton dipped in tea. The combination helped to prevent infection. After three to four weeks of using it, the tear duct opened and was able to drain.

### Fasting Combination

1. _____ Licorice, Beet Root, Hawthorne Berries, Fennel Seed.
   — helps give energy and controls hunger while fasting.

### *Case History:*

Whenever N. tried to go on a juice fast she got headaches. She tried using 6 capsules a day of Fasting Combination when she went on a fast and had no more headaches.

### Female Corrective Combinations

1. _____ Goldenseal, Red Raspberry, Black Cohosh, Queen of the Meadows, Marshmallow, Blessed Thistle, Lobelia, Capsicum, Ginger.

2. _____ Red Raspberry Leaves, Dong Quai, Ginger, Licorice, Black Cohosh, Queen of the Meadow, Blessed Thistle, Marshmallow.

3. _____ Goldenseal, Blessed Thistle, Capsicum,

Uva Ursi, Cramp Bark, False Unicorn, Red Raspberry, Squaw Vine, Ginger.

4. _____ Black Cohosh, Sarsaparilla, Ginseng, Licorice, False Unicorn, Blessed Thistle, Squawvine.

— contain female hormones that help regulate the female system, normalize menstrual periods and stop menstrual cramps or any uterine problem.

— helps with acne in young girls if it is caused by a hormonal imbalance.

— been used before, during and after pregnancy. Also used to prevent morning sickness and miscarriages.

— when taken with Red Raspberry tea it helps to stimulate ovulation in infertility problems.

— used for hot flashes and problems of menopause. Especially Female Corrective Combination #4.

NOTE: Start with small amount and work up to needed dosage gradually.

MOST COMMON USES

| | | |
|---|---|---|
| Acne | Menopause | Pregnancy |
| Female Problems | Menstrual Cramps | Puberty |
| Hot Flashes | Morning Sickness | Sterility |
| Infertility | Nausea | Uterine Problems |
| Lymphatic System | Ovulation | |

### Case History:

A woman in her 20's not only had problems with extreme heavy menstrual flow, but also had debilitating cramps as well. She had been to many doctors and specialists and had taken many kinds of prescriptions. They had found a prescription that worked for the pain; she took it for a few years until it was taken off the market. She tried Bayberry and a nerve combination with the next period and experienced relief from the heavy flow, but not from the pain. She took six capsules Female Formula #1 a day through the following month. When her period started she added 1-2 capsules Bayberry for the heavy flow and a herbal pain relieving formula. She was able to stay at her job during her period for the first time in years.

Each month brought more improvement. She continues to take the female formula #1 everyday but no longer adds extra Bayberry because the heavy flow has stopped. She plans to continue taking the female formula until the problem is corrected.

## Flu Combinations

1. _____ Ginger, Capsicum, Goldenseal, Licorice.

2. _____ Bayberry Bark, Ginger, White Pine Bark, Capsicum, Clove Powder.

— Clove tea helps with cramps and diarrhea of flu. (See Baby Chapter.) Goldenseal is an infection fighter, licorice soothes inflamed mucous membranes. Ginger helps with nausea.

— these combination also combat secondary infections.

MOST COMMON USES

| | | |
|---|---|---|
| Aches of flu | Flu-Influenza | Sinus problems |
| Colds | Head colds | Stomach ache |
| Cramps, flu | Infection | Throat, sore |
| Diarrhea | Menstrual Cramping | Vomiting |
| Fever | Nausea, including air & car sickness | |

*Case History:*

M. started using the Flu Combination #1 for the flu. At first she noticed the flu was just lasting less time than her neighbors. 1 to 3 days instead of 7-14. Then she found if she gave a dose at the very start of the flu, that most of the time the person never got the flu. Sometimes only one dose was necessary. Even if they came down with the flu, it didn't last very long and the symptoms weren't as severe as before. By doing this she and her family went through a whole winter with flu all around them without ever succumbing to it; except for one family member who didn't take the combination. (See Flu-Influenza in Ailments chapter)

## General Cleanser and Parasites Combination

1. _____ Gentian, Irish Moss, Goldenseal, Comfrey, Fenugreek Seeds, Mandrake, Safflower, Myrrh Gum, Yellow Dock, Echinacea, Black Walnut, Barberry, Dandelion, St. Johnswort, Chickweed, Catnip, Cyani.

— used to cleanse the body of cysts, tumors, parasites, mucus, etc.

— should be taken with an herbal laxative or enemas.

— kills parasites anywhere in the body, even malaria parasite. For malaria parasite, some people add an extra capsule of Black Walnut.

— pinworms are usually infested in the appendix as well as the colon. The prescription drug for pinworms only cleans the intestines.

— after the first bottle, another bottle should be repeated in 4-5 weeks to kill any eggs that might have hatched. Adults have taken 3-6 a day and children, about 1 a day.

### Case History

J. took one capsule three times a day until the bottle of 100 capsules was gone and passed dead parasites every day for four months.

### Parasite Combination

1. _____ Pumpkin Seeds, Culvers Root, Mandrake, Violet Leaves, Poke Root, Cascara Sagrada, Witch Hazel, Mullein, Comfrey, Slippery Elm.
   — used for parasites and prostate problems. (Many times prostate problems are related to parasites in the colon close to the prostate.)
   — some people take this combination for parasites after finding that General Cleanser and Parasites Combination #1 cleanses too fast and gives them a headache.
   — contains pumpkin seeds which contain zinc. Zinc is good for prostate problems and also kills parasites.
   — contains cascara sagrada, an herbal laxative to help move toxins out of the body. Extra cascara sagrada or (another herbal laxative) may be necessary.
MOST COMMON USES
Prostate                    Worms-parasites,
                                       expels

### Glandular Combination

1. _____ Mullein, Lobelia.
   — used for glandular swelling and malfunctioning glands.
MOST COMMON USES
Glands

### Hair, Skin and Nails Combination or Mineral Combinations

1. _____ Kelp, Dandelion, Alfalfa.

2. _____ Dulse, Horsetail, Sage, Rosemary.
   — high in minerals for improvement in hair, skin, and nails.
   — #1 is also used for dogs to improve their coat and health.
   — #1 is used by pregnant women because it contains kelp, and herbs high in minerals.

— prevents and removes white spots on nails.
MOST COMMON USES

| Anemia | Hair | Minerals |
|--------|------|----------|
| Nails | Pregnancy | Skin |

## Headache and Pain Combinations

1. _____ Valerian Root, Wild Lettuce, Capsicum.
— used for stress or nervous headaches. Valerian Root is very healing and soothing to nervous system.
— very good for arthritis pain-has been taken as often as every two hours-4-6 capsules.
— also used for afterpains after childbirth and for menstrual cramps.
— general pain reliever anywhere in the body, sore throats, earaches, etc. Wild lettuce and Valerian Root are both pain relieving herbs.
— comes in capsules and extract.
MOST COMMON USES

| Afterpain, childbirth | Headache | Stress |
|---|---|---|
| Arthritis | Heartpain | Throat, sore |
| Cramps, menstrual | Nerves | |
| Earache | Pain | |

### Case History

— Anytime C gets any aches or pains including those caused by flu or even leg aches-she takes anywhere from 2 to 6 capsules of Headache and Pain Combination as needed and gets relief. She also used it for afterpains after childbirth. She took 4 capsules as needed for pain. There was no problem with afterpain and she never had to take a drug pain reliever. Headache and Pain Combination #1 is one to keep on hand for all kind of stress or pain.

## Headache Combination

1. _____ Fenugreek, Thyme.
— used with good success for migraine headaches. Helps stop the pounding, throbbing and the nausea (see remedies.)
— has calming action on nerves.
— also helps sinus headache pain and helps pull mucus from whole body.

MOST COMMON USES

Migraine headaches      Mucus, in head       Sinus

## *Case History*

— M. had frequent headaches. She hadn't found anything to help the pain except powerful drugs. Pain relieving herbs had not helped either until she learned about Fenugreek and Thyme in combination. She tried it with her next migraine. She took six capsules every 2-3 hours for three days until her headache was gone. She was able to function quite normally instead of lying in bed.

## Infection Fighting Combinations

1. _____ Rose Hips Powder, Chamomile, Slippery Elm, Yarrow, Capsicum, Goldenseal, Myrrh Gum, Peppermint, Sage, Lemon Grass.

2. _____ Echinacea, Goldenseal, Yarrow, Capsicum.

3. _____ Echinacea, Yarrow, Myrrh, Capsicum.

4. _____ Plantain, Black Walnut, Goldenseal, Bugleweed, Marshmallow, Lobelia.

5. _____ Garlic, Rosehips, Parsley, Watercress.

6. _____ Garlic, Capsicum.

7. _____ Chickweed, Black Cohosh, Goldenseal, Lobelia, Skullcap, Brigham Tea, Licorice.
   — for amounts that have been used see Colds and Acute Illness, Ailments Chapter.
   — fights infection and contain natural antibiotics.
   — kills bacteria and virus, all types of infections.
   — works with the friendly bacteria, doesn't destroy it. Since friendly bacteria is a natural defense mechanism, the body is stronger in fighting infection.
   — stimulates the body to heal itself.
   — reduces fevers.
   — helps sleep and relaxation.
   — pulls toxins, has diuretic properties.
   — moves mucus out of the body so no need for antihistamines.
   — infection fighting combinations #2 and #3 are the same except

that Myrrh has been substituted for Goldenseal in #3. Because of the Goldenseal, #3 is used by some hypoglycemics instead of #2.

MOST COMMON USES

| | | |
|---|---|---|
| Allergies | Flu-Influenza | Mucus |
| Bronchitis | Head Colds | Pneumonia |
| Earaches | Infections | Prostate |
| Ear Infections | Insect Bites, Stings | Sinus |
| Emphysema | Kidney Infections | Throat, Sore |
| Fevers | Lymph Glands | Tonsillitis |

*Case History:*

I have used these infection fighting combinations with my family of six children for sore throats, tonsillitis, swollen glands, earaches, bronchitis and respiratory problems, kidney infections, flu, etc . . . I haven't needed to use a synthetic antibiotic for fourteen years.

**Infertility and Impotency Combination**

1. _____ Ginseng, Echinacea, Saw Palmetto, Gota Kola, Damiana, Sarsaparilla, Periwinkle, Garlic, Capsicum, Chickweed.

— contains both male and female hormones and has been used to regulate and stimulate the reproductive organs.

— contains cayenne and ginseng so it stimulates energy.

— some miscarriages are caused by women not having enough hormones. The Progesterone hormone helps the uterus prepare for a pregnancy so it can carry a baby.

MOST COMMON USES

| | | |
|---|---|---|
| Endurance | Hot Flashes | Miscarriage |
| Energy | Impotency | Senility |
| Frigidity | Longevity | Sex Stimulant |
| Hormones | Menopause | Sterility |

*Case History:*

A man was having impotency problems. He tried the Infertility, Impotency Combination, after 2 weeks the impotency problem was much improved.

This combination has also helped men who have impotency problems because of spinal injuries.

### Intestinal Cleanser Combination

1. _____ Comfrey, Pepsin.

Eating lots of refined foods coats the lining of the small intestine with a mucus film. This mucus film doesn't allow the nutrients to pass through the small intestines efficiently so the individual does not receive proper nourishment from their food. Pepsin, a digestive enzyme, aids in the digestion of this unwanted mucus film. Comfrey is sticky and holds the pepsin to the intestinal wall long enough to digest this film of mucus. Dr. William D. Kelly made the statement that if he only had one pill to take, this combination would be it.

— Taken for three to four months, it helps to digest the mucous film, so better assimilation can take place.

— Once the film is gone it is a good idea to take this combination once a year for 3 to 4 weeks to keep the intestinal lining from becoming coated again.

— is also a general digestive aid and tones the small intestine and colon.

MOST COMMON USES

| | | |
|---|---|---|
| Colon, tones | Mucus | Small Intestine |
| Digestion | | |

### Kidney and Bladder Combinations

1. _____ Juniper Berries, Parsley, Uva Ursi leaves, Dandelion Root, Chamomile.

2. _____ Juniper Berries, Parsley, Uva Ursi, Marshmallow, Lobelia, Ginger, Goldenseal.

— acts as a diuretic, helps cleanse, heal and normalize the kidneys, bladder and urinary passages.

— good for infections of the kidney and bladder especially when used with the infection fighting combinations.

— taken one hour before bedtime has helped bedwetting problems.

— helps dissolve kidney stones.

— safe to use as a diuretic during pregnancy for swelling and water retention.

— have also been used in place of diuretic drugs (for high blood pressure, water retention, etc.) NOTE: The herbs in these combinations are rich in potassium so they do not deplete the body of potassium as diuretic drugs do.

MOST COMMON USES

| | | |
|---|---|---|
| Bedwetting | Diuretic | Pregnancy Diuretic |
| Bladder, infections | Kidneys | Water Retention |
| and problems | Kidney Stones | |

### *Case History:*

B. had a kidney infection. He even had blood in his urine. He took this combination along with the infection fighting combination and it completely cleared up in three to four days.

### Liver/Gall Bladder Combinations

1. _____ Red Beet Root, Dandelion, Parsley Herb, Horsetail, Liverworst, Birch Leaves, Lobelia, Blessed Thistle, Angelica Root, Chamomile, Gentian, Goldenrod.

2. _____ Barberry Bark, Cramp Bark, Fennel, Ginger, Catnip, Peppermint, Wild Yam.

### *Liver*

The liver has been called the waste disposal or detoxification organ. One of its jobs is to purify poisonous substances from the blood. It is a filtering organ. Many drugs and minerals in unassimilable forms (inorganic iron etc.) end up stored in the liver.

The liver can also become infected, jaundiced, obstructed and have cancer. This combination helps the liver to cleanse, heal and function normally.

### *Gall Bladder*

The liver manufactures bile, a digestive secretion; the gall bladders stores and excretes it into the small intestine when needed. These combinations help the gall bladder function normally and prevent gall stones.

MOST COMMON USES

| | | |
|---|---|---|
| Age spots (liverspots) | Hepatitis | Spleen |
| Gall Bladder | Liver | Yellow Jaundice |

### Lower Bowel Combinations

1. _____ Cascara Sagrada, Buckthorn, Licorice

Root, Capsicum, Ginger, Barberry, Couch Grass, Red Clover, Lobelia.

2. _____ Cascara Sagrada, Barberry Bark, Capsicum, Ginger, Lobelia, Red Raspberry, Golden Seal, Fennel, Turkey Rhubarb.

— good for constipation, normalizes colon function, is not habit forming.

— tones bowel tissue and stimulates peristaltic action, not an irritant to the bowel.

— expels parasites and mucus from the pockets in colon.

— also good for colitis problems.

MOST COMMON USES

| | | |
|---|---|---|
| Bowel Function | Constiptation | Peristaltic Action |
| Colitis | Diverticulitis | Worms-Parasites, expels. |

## Lung Combinations

1. _____ Comfrey, Mullein, Marshmallow, Lobelia, Slippery Elm.

2. _____ Comfrey, Fenugreek.

3. _____ Marshmallow, Mullein, Lobelia, Chickweed.

— helps to expel mucus from the lungs.

— used to quiet coughing spasms, especially #1 and #3.

— helps stop chest pain due to cough, bronchitis or pneumonia.

— fights infection, best results in fighting infections are achieved when used with an infection fighting combination. (See Ailments)

MOST COMMON USES

| | | |
|---|---|---|
| Asthma | Hay Fever | Pain in chest, |
| Bronchitis | Hoarseness | due to lung |
| Coughs | Lungs | infections |
| Emphysema | Mucus, in lungs | Pleurisy |
| | | Pneumonia |

### *Case History:*

A. had had a residual cough left over from a cold. He was unable to sleep because he kept coughing all night. He had never used herbs but his wife had. Finally, one night his wife gave him 6 capsules of

Lung Combination #2. He slept through the night without cough-ing. He took 6 capsules 4 times a day for two days, 4 capsules 4 times a day for two days, and then 3 capsules 4 times a day for two more days. The cough was gone.

Another lady had coughing that caused intense chest pain. She didn't have anything on hand to take except for Lung Combination #1. She took 4 capsules every few hours, the chest pain left. The coughing eased and was gone in a few days.

## Nerve and Relaxing Combinations

1. _____ Valerian Root, Wild Lettuce, Capsicum.

2. _____ Black Cohosh, Capsicum, Valerian Root, Mistletoe, Ginger Root, St. Johnswort, Hops, Wood Betony.

3. _____ Valerian Root, Skullcap, Hops.

4. _____ Black Cohosh, Capsicum, Hops, Mis-tletoe, Lobelia, Scullcap, Wood Betony, Lady Slipper, Valerian Root.
   — calms nerves.

### Why Nerve and Relaxing Combinations

Mental stress and tension cause the nerves to become tired and worn down. Also most biological problems are related to stress. The nerve herbs feed and strengthen the nerves so one can handle stress better. The nerve herbs also have a calming, quieting effect on the nerves. These combinations are good to have on hand for times when one is under any kind of stress.
MOST COMMON USES

| | | |
|---|---|---|
| Arthritis | Headache | Smoking |
| Asthma | Hypoglycemia | Stress |
| Diabetes | Insomnia-sleep | |
| | Nerves | |

### Case History:

A. had a glandular imbalance because of a low functioning pitui-tary gland. This imbalance caused her to be very nervous. She took 2 to 4 capsules of the Nerve Combination #1 every 4 hours or when she started feeling nervous. It gave her a calm feeling. She eventu-ally was able to cut down on the nerve combination until she didn't need it anymore.

## Pancreas Combinations

1. _____ Goldenseal, Juniper Berries, Uva Ursi, Huckleberry Leaves, Mullein, Comfrey, Yarrow, Garlic, Capsicum, Dandelion, Marshmallow, Buchu, Bistort, Licorice. (Diabetes)

2. _____ Cedar Berries, Uva Ursi, Licorice, Mullein, Capsicum, Goldenseal.

3. _____ Licorice Root, Safflower Flowers, Dandelion Root, Horseradish Root. (Hypoglycemia)

— helps both the adrenals and pancreas glands to heal and function normally.

— the *pancreas* secretes insulin into the blood stream. *Hypo*glycemia or low blood sugar is caused by the pancreas constantly supplying too much insulin. Diabetes or *Hyper*glycemia high blood sugar is caused when the pancreas can no longer supply enough insulin for the sugar intake.

— many people think diabetes and hypoglycemia are two different diseases, when they are in fact stages of the same disease, with Hypoglycemia the start of diabetes.

— in hypoglycemia, the pancreas is injured or becoming damaged so it behaves erratically. This helps to explain the highs and lows of hypoglycemia. As the hypoglycemic eats food, especially food high in sugars, the blood sugar rises; the pancreas panics and releases too much insulin. This causes the blood sugar to fall drastically. The uneducated hypoglycemic will then feel a need for more sugar and eat it and the cycle will be repeated with high/low, high/low. Over a period of time the pancreas will cease to produce insulin. At this stage the hypoglycemic starts to switch over to a diabetic.

— in diabetes, the sugar road has been traveled a little further. In the case of juvenile diabetes, a pancreas weakness may have been received at birth. However, in some cases parasites in the isle of pancreas, or viral disease injuring the pancreas may be the cause. At any rate, in diabetes, the pancreas is extremely damaged and in some cases not functioning at all. Diabetics, like all people with chronic problems, need to realize that it took time to get where they are and it is going to take time to get back. Proper diet, exercise, knowledge of their own body and a positive mental attitude combined with the pancreas and adrenal herbs are extremely important for managing diabetes.

NOTE: The statement was once made by a person that Hypoglycemia was the most over-diagnosed disease. With the eating habits of the typical American, perhaps it is the most **under**-diagnosed disease. No, what you feel is not all in your head.

— The *adrenal glands* control the secretion of adrenalin which helps with energy levels, blood sugar, rate and force of the heart beat, oxygen consumption and heat production and in helping skeletal muscles to cope with emergencies. The adrenal glands usually start to become affected before the pancreas. One reason why the hypoglycemic and diabetic find it tiring and difficult to exercise is because of the lack of sufficient adrenalin. Healthy adrenal glands are necessary for an energetic and vital life.

MOST COMMON USES

| | | |
|---|---|---|
| Adrenal Glands | Diabetes | Pancreas |
| Blood Sugar Problems | Hypoglycemia | |

## Poultice Combinations

1. _____ Comfrey, Goldenseal, Slippery Elm, Aloe Vera

— used for infections of any kind internal or external.

— pulls slivers, rocks, etc. from scraped or embedded flesh wounds (Poultice)

— has cell proliferation action so helps heal wounds quickly.

— contains natural pain relievers. Relieves soreness cuts and wounds.

— for poultice, mix with mineral water or aloe vera juice or gel and add either vitamin E oil, castor oil, or olive oil and apply directly on wound (see remedies.)

— used to take pain and swelling from broken limbs, sprains or infected sores (poultice.)

— excellent results when used for hiatal hernia or ulcers. Mix with a little water and drink so it will coat the area. The results are well worth its bitter taste.

— good to have on hand for any kinds of wounds, scrapes, slivers, etc.

MOST COMMON USES

| | | |
|---|---|---|
| Blood poisoning | Inflammation | Wounds |
| Cuts | Insect bites, stings | Wounds, puncture |
| Hiatal hernia | Sores | |
| Infection, external or internal | Swellings | |
| | Ulcers | |

*Case History:*

G., a child had a puncture wound on her heel. It became very swollen and red until the child could not walk. Poultice #1 was applied and within a half hour, the child was running around playing. Another poultice was applied 24 hours later. It was the last one applied because the puncture wound healed very rapidly. The case histories on this combination could fill a book, it is a very valuable combination.

## Broken Bone Poultice Combination

2. _____ Comfrey, White Oak Bark, Mullein, Black Walnut, Marshmallow, Queen of the Meadow, Wormwood, Lobelia, Scullcap.
   — used to help heal broken bones, ligaments and joints.
   — a good poultice for quick healing of healing bones; supplies much calcium.
   MOST COMMON USES

| | | |
|---|---|---|
| Broken bones | Joints | Ligaments |
| Gout | | |

## Pre-Natal Combinations

1. _____ Black Cohosh, Squawvine, Lobelia, Penny Royal, Red Raspberries.

2. _____ Squawvine, Blessed Thistle, Black Cohosh, False Unicorn, Pennyroyal, Red Raspberry, Lobelia.
   — has been used for the last five weeks of pregnancy.
   — strengthens and tones uterus, promotes easier labor.
   — taking this formula and Blue Cohosh together the last five weeks during pregnancy is especially effective for those who have problems with the cervix dialating. (See Pregnancy chapter)
   — can be taken after delivery.
   MOST COMMON USES—Labor

*Case History:*

R. always had long drawn-out labors. She used the Prenatal Combination #1 and had three hours of labor instead of 17. She recommends this combination to others and has used it for subsequent pregnancies.
A., had her fifth child at 40 years of age. After using the pre-natal

combination during this pregnancy, she was told by her doctor at her six week check-up that her uterus looked as good as if she had never been pregnant.

## Prostate Combinations

1. _____ Black Cohosh, Licorice Root, Kelp, Gotu Kola, Capsicum, Ginger Root, Lobelia, Goldenseal.

2. _____ Capsicum, Uva Ursi, Parsley, Goldenseal, Gravel Root, Juniper Berries, Marshmallow, Ginger, Ginseng.
   — cleanses prostate gland.
   — prostate cancer is becoming more prevalent. Cleansing this gland should help prevent this.
   — expels blood, old cellular material, and toxins from urinary tract in many cases. Then healing can take place.
   — contains both male and female hormones.
   MOST COMMON USES

| Hormones | Prostate | Urinary problems |
|---|---|---|

*Case History:*

J. an adult male started having problems with pain in the prostate area and bedwetting at night. After taking the prostate combination for a few days, he passed a lot of debris and also broke out in a rash in the area. He took garlic enemas along with the combination to help carry toxins out of the system. After this he had no more problems with pain or urination at night.

## Protein Combinations

1. _____ Soy protein, Capsicum, Red Clover.
   — used as a pickup for hypoglycemics.
   — gives assimilable protein in a capsule.
   — the cayenne also acts as an energy booster and as a catalyst for the protein.
   MOST COMMON USE-Hypoglycemia

## Thyroid Combinations

1. _____ Kelp, Irish Moss, Parsley, Capsicum.

2. _____ Parsley, Watercress, Kelp, Irish Moss, Black Walnut, Sarsaparilla, Iceland Moss.

— regulates the thyroid gland whether hyper-thyroid (over active) or hypo-thyroid (under active.)

— when synthetic thyroxin goes into the blood stream it tells the thyroid there is already thyroxin in the blood thus the thyroid ceases to function.normally.

— herbs for the thyroid aid the thyroid so it can regulate itself and produce the thyroxin the body needs.

— contains nutrients and minerals, including iodine and trace minerals, that feed the thyroid.

— helps to regulate body temperature.

MOST COMMON USES

| | | |
|---|---|---|
| Allergies | Epilepsy | Obesity |
| Digestion | Goiter | Thyroid |
| Diuretic | Iodine | |
| Energy | Minerals | |

### *Case History:*

B. had an underactive thyroid. She tried synthetic thyroxin for a while and then changed to the Thyroid combination #1. Within a few months, her thyroid was functioning so well that she no longer needed the herbal combination for her thyroid. This response is not unusual. **(The herbs seem to try to put themselves out of a job whereas many times drugs cause the body to depend upon them.)**

### Ulcer Combination

1. _____ Goldenseal, Capsicum, Myrrh.
   — "contact healers," they also help stop bleeding.
   — works throughout the entire digestive system.
   — adding Slippery Elm makes an even more soothing formula.
   — used as a tea to rinse the mouth for cankers or sore gums.
   — drink tea or stir powder in water for hiatal hernia.
   MOST COMMON USES

| | | |
|---|---|---|
| Cankers | Colitis | Gums, sore (tea) |
| Hiatal Hernia | Sores, in mouth | Ulcers |

### *Case History:*

D. suffered with ulcers for years. He took 2 capsules of this combination a half hour before meals and in a short time he was able to eat fresh vegetables and other formerly forbidden foods again.

**Vaginal Bolus**

1. _____ Squawvine, Chickweed, Slippery Elm
   — used to cleanse the uterine and vaginal area.
   — has helped dissolve cysts on ovaries. (see remedies, Women Only Chapter.)
   — adding goldenseal to this combination makes it even more effective.
   — comes in powdered bulk form. For instructions on making bolus see "Other Remedies" in For Women only.
   MOST COMMON USES

| | | |
|---|---|---|
| Endometriosis | Ovarian cysts | Vagina |
| Leucorrhea | Uterine cancer | |

**Weight Loss Combination**

1. _____ Chickweed, Mandrake, Licorice, Safflowers, Echinacea, Black Walnut Hulls, Gota Kola, Hawthorne Berries, Papaya, Fennel Seed, Dandelion.
   — aids in normalizing glands and brings them back in balance.
   — decreases the appetite and aids in digestion, some people add extra chickweed for more weight loss.
   — acts as a general cleanser and as a laxative to carry out the toxins.
   — gives energy.
   — acts as a diuretic.
   NOTE: Since this combination is a general cleanser, large doses of this are not needed nor recommended. Adults should take no more than 6 capsules a day. Start with 1 capsule a day and work up.
   MOST COMMON USES

| | | |
|---|---|---|
| Constipation | Diuretic | Worms-Parasites, |
| during weight | Energy | expels. |
| loss | General Cleanser | Weight Loss |

*Case History:*

M., lost 50 pounds on this combination. She felt good, had a lot of energy and was not constipated. She had a good mental attitude while losing weight because she felt good. She had no problems with water retention.

Her husband noticed how happy she seemed. He said he didn't care what she was taking, but to keep on taking it.

# CHAPTER 3

# Vitamins and Minerals

## VITAMINS AND MINERALS

Vitamins and minerals are included in this book because using them with herbs causes a **synergistic** relationship. That means the parts work together so they enhance and complement each other. The total effect becomes greater than the total of the individual effects. And, also, because herbs contain vitamins and minerals. Learning about vitamins and minerals will help you to better understand the properties of herbs. Vitamins, minerals, and herbs are more effective when used together against disease and problems than when used separately. In the Ailment Chapter, specific herbs and vitamins will be suggested for different ailments.

## VITAMINS

In order for a substance to be defined as a vitamin it must be essential for life. Plants manufacture their own vitamins, but animal bodies usually do not; therefore, we must obtain them from an outside source, either in the food we eat or through a supplement.

If we ate only raw, fresh food that has been grown organically in fertile soil, we probably wouldn't need supplements. (Note: Some foods require cooking to make them palatable and assimilable, but a majority of our foods are "cooked to death.") Because of the "instant" age in which we live overprocessed and overcooked foods, unwise food habits, and unreplenished soil deplete the vitamins (and minerals) in the food we eat.

In *The Complete Book of Vitamins* by the Staff of Prevention Magazine we read:

> "According to Jean Mayer, Ph.D., of Harvard's School of Public Health (Science, 21 April 1972), in 1941 only 10 percent of our foods were highly processed. 'Today,' he wrote, 'that amount has risen to 50 percent.' And while processing of food has increased so drastically chronic, degenerative disease has increased too."

Somehow suspecting a relationship between eating a decrease of whole unprocessed food and the increase of degenerative diseases does not seem unrealistic, especially in light of the recent findings of researchers.

Vitamins act as preventatives by keeping the body strong, able to defend against disease. Vitamins build, strengthen and nourish the body.

## VITAMIN DEFICIENCY

Note: Individual vitamin deficiencies are discussed later in this chapter under each of the individual vitamins.

The diseases scurvy and rickets come to mind when vitamin deficiencies are discussed because of the great trouble they caused until the cure was found. It is our belief that many problems are caused by a lack of a vitamin, a mineral or a nutrient and that some of these deficiencies are as yet unrecognized or unbelieved by a great part of our society. It is possible to help a health problem by adding or increasing a certain vitamin or mineral. As more research is being done, the significance adequate vitamins and minerals play in good health is being realized.

## VITAMIN ASSIMILATION

— Synthetic vitamins are the pure vitamin with nothing added. These vitamins are "created" by man. Natural vitamins are the whole vitamins from a natural source. In 1977 approximately 15 vitamins had been discovered and scientists believed that twice as many as that may exist. By 1980 scientists had identified at least 20 vitamins. In the space of approximately 80 years man had "discovered" 20 plus vitamins, but mother nature has known about them all along-and she knows the ones that remain unidentified. She has been putting them in her food for years.

— A second reason in favor of natural vitamins is because the natural vitamin, being whole, has elements in it that help the body to assimilate the vitamins. Often synthetic vitamins are in a form that the body is unable to break down, so they simply pass through the system without being used. If our health isn't good we may have digestion problems. It makes sense to take vitamins in a form that is easiest to assimilate. The most expensive vitamins are the ones that are not assimilated. (The other expensive vitamins are the ones that sit in the bottle stored in the cupboard, while their shelf life decreases.)

Find good natural vitamins with a base of yeast or herbs which help assimilation of the vitamins. Vitamins of this type, whether they are capsuled or pressed into a tablet usually contain herbs or enzymes to help assimilation of the vitamins.

## DIFFERENT APPROACHES TO VITAMINS

In *The Complete Book of Vitamins* by the Staff of Prevention Magazine three ways that people take vitamins are reported.

### 1. "Insurance method or approach."

People who use this idea take only enough of each vitamin each day to insure against a deficiency disease. They follow closely the Recommended Daily Allowance for each vitamin. This is the most common form of vitamin-usage and was started out of fear of the horrible deficiency diseases.

### 2. Maximum positive benefits approach.

This method suggests using the amount the body needs to obtain maximum health without taking huge doses. People who use this approach really do feel better. Many diseases *not* normally associated with vitamins have been reduced by using this method.

### 3. Mega-vitamin therapy.

This method uses large amounts of vitamins instead of drugs to fight disease. The results achieved with megavitamin therapy are remarkable. See Mega-Vitamin Therapy this chapter.

For more information see *The Complete Book of Vitamins* pp. 67-76. Also *Dr. Wright's Book of Nutritional Therapy* by Jonathan V. Wright M.D. is a book that tells of Dr. Wright's treatment of diseases with vitamins and minerals.

## HOW TO TAKE VITAMINS

Recommended Daily Allowances and Minimum Daily Allowances (RDA and MDA) will not be put in this book. They are just recommendations for the average person, and there is no "average" person.

1.  Take a natural multiple vitamin and mineral supplement as a **foundation** for vitamin taking *and then* if one has the need add extra single vitamins and minerals. This also applies to the B Vitamins, a B Complex should be taken and then any extra single B's can be added with it. We need the whole circle of vitamins for them to be as effective as possible. A multiple also helps in assimilation of the extra single ones.

If we make sure that we get the minimum foundation of vitamins and minerals each day, we have a better chance of preventing or throwing off illness when it enters our body.

2.  Take supplements with a meal. Breakfast is a good suggestion for this since it is the start of the day's activity. Taking vitamins with a meal will help assimilation. Some people use digestive enzymes to aid assimilation.

3.  Space water soluble vitamins by taking them at different times throughout the day. This way the body is able to use more of the vitamin rather than just excreting the excess.

## MEGA-VITAMIN THERAPY

Vitamins are like herbs in that there are infection fighting vitamins, vitamins that promote hormonal balance, vitamins that work as natural antihistamines, ones that are cancer deterrents, vitamins for skin problems, bruises, wound healing, ulcers and any number of ailments. When trying to help an ailment we switch to mega-vitamin therapy using the Infection Fighting Vitamins-A, C, and E.

The following is what we use for colds, coughs, ear aches, sore throats, any acute illness.

|                                               | **Adults**              | **Children 12-16**      |
| --------------------------------------------- | ----------------------- | ----------------------- |
| Multiple Vitamin and Mineral Supplement       | 1                       | 1                       |
| Vitamin A                                     | 100,000 I.U./day        | 75,000 I.U./day         |
| Vitamin C                                     | 1,000 mg. every 2-3 hours | 1,000 mg. every 2-3 hours |
| Vitamin E                                     | 400 I.U./day            | 200 I.U./day            |

|                                               | **Children 6-12**       | **Children 3-6**        |
| --------------------------------------------- | ----------------------- | ----------------------- |
| Multiple Vitamin and Mineral Supplement       | 1                       | 1                       |
| Vitamin A                                     | 25-50,000 I.U./day      | 10-20,000 I.U./day      |
| Vitamin C                                     | 1,000 mg. every 2-3 hours | 1,000 mg. every 2-3 hours |
| Vitamin E                                     | 100 I.U./day            | 100 I.U./day            |

We use these infection fighting vitamins along with the infection fighting herbs.

For allergies and sore throats we use the above combinations and add:

|                  | **Adults**            | **Children 12-16**    |
| ---------------- | --------------------- | --------------------- |
| B Complex        | 1                     | 1                     |
| Pantothenic Acid | 100 mg. every 4 hours | 100 mg. every 4 hours |

|                                             | **Children 6-12**   | **Children 3-6**    |
| ------------------------------------------- | ------------------- | ------------------- |
| Children's Multiple Vitamin high in B Complex | 1                 | 1                   |
| Pantothenic Acid                            | 50 mg. every 4 hours | 25 mg. every 4 hours |

Note: Vitamins for Babies—See Baby Chapter

# INDIVIDUAL VITAMINS

## VITAMIN A (RETINOL, CAROTENE)

Fat soluble. Essential for the body to manufacture visual purple, which is necessary for night vision. Vitamin A requires fats as well as minerals to be assimilated. Vitamin A is an **antioxidant**. Antioxidants protect other substances from uncontrolled oxidations that damage cells. They help keep pollutants in check. (Antioxidants are A, C, E, and Selenium)

**Positive Effects**

Strengthens weak eyesight

Healthy skin

Acne

Corrects Blackheads

Impetigo

Boils

Carbuncles

Open ulcers

Keeps outer layers or organs and tissues healthy

Hair

Teeth and gums

Builds resistance to disease

Aids in treatment of emphysema and hyperthyroidism

Respiratory infections

Hay Fever, allergies

Anti-cancer agent

Strong bones

Promotes growth

Delays senility

Prolongs longevity

Aids in protein digestion

Offsets affects of pollution

**Deficiency Disease-**Xerophthalmia (night blindness)

**Signs of Deficiency**

Eye disorders

Red, itchy eyes

Rough or goose bumpy skin

Dry, brittle hair

Poor growth in young

Susceptibility to infection

Loss of appetite and weight

Sterility

Impaired sense of smell

**Toxicity-**As a fat soluble vitamin A can be toxic if overdosed. However, adults have safely taken 100,000 I.U. daily and infants have safely taken 18,000 I.U. daily for many months.

**Enemies-**Modern interior lighting, polyunsaturated fatty acids with carotene unless antioxidants are present.

**Natural Sources-**Fish, butter, carrots, yellow vegetables, very green vegetables, liver, eggs, whole milk, fish liver oil, yellow fruits.

**Herb Sources-**Alfalfa, Black Cohosh, Bee Pollen, Burdock, Capsicum, Catnip, Camomile, Comfrey, Dandelion, Dong Quai, Echinacea, Eyebright, Fennel, Fenugreek, Garlic, Ginger, Ginseng, Goldenseal, Kelp, Marshmallow, Mullein, Papaya, Peppermint, Poke Root, Red Clover, Red Raspberry, Rose Hips, Rosemary, Sage, Sarsaparilla, Saw Palmetto, Yarrow, Yellow Dock.

# VITAMIN B₁ (THIAMINE)

Water soluble. Also called **morale or pep** vitamins. All B vitamins should be taken with a B complex.

## Positive Effects

Improves mental attitude
Prevents premature aging
Protein and Carbohydrate
    metabolism
Appetite stabilization
Improves digestion
Helps fight air or seasickness
Reduces edema
Mild diuretic
Prevention of excessive
    fatty deposits on wall arteries

Maintains normal red blood
    count
Good muscle tone of heart,
    intestines, and stomach
Growth in children
Relieves pain after dental
    work
Prevents Beri-Beri
Shingles
Antioxidant

## Deficiency Disease-Beri-Beri
## Signs of Deficiency

Memory loss
Mental confusion
Emotional instability
Irritability
Loss of mental alertness
Central nervous system problems
Brain damamge
Numb hands and feet

Pains around heart and nerves
Heart function irregularities
Shortness of breath
Fatigue
Loss of appetite
Gastro-intestinal discomfort
    and pain
Constipation
Weight loss

**Toxicity-**none known.

**Enemies-**cooking, heat, caffeine, alcohol, food processing methods, air, water, estrogen, sulfa drugs, sugar.

**Natural Sources-**wheat bran, brewers yeast, wheat germ, whole grains, nuts, eggs, beef, pork, lamb, turkey, organ meats, fish, blackstrap molasess, brown rice, beets, leafy green vegetables, potatoes.

**Herb Sources-**Alfalfa, Blue Cohosh, Burdock, Capsicum, Cascara, Catnip, Chickweed, Dandelion, Eyebright, Fenugreek, Garlic, Ginger, Goldenseal, Hawthorne, Hops, Kelp, Licorice, Marshmallow, Mullein, Papaya, Red Clover.

## VITAMIN B₂ (RIBOFLAVIN)

Called the youth vitamin. Water soluble. Not destroyed by heat, oxidation or acid. Increased need for it during stress. **Most common vitamin deficiency in America is Vitamin B₂.** Much riboflavin in milk is destroyed by the light used to create Vitamin D in milk.

### Positive Effects

Stress

Promotes healthy skin, nails
  and hair

Aids in growth and reproduction

Helps prevent birth abnormalities

Helps failing vision in
  final weeks of preganancy

Aids in absorption of iron

Relieves burning sensations
  of hands and feet

Benefits vision and eye
  fatigue

Helps certain kinds of cataracts

Helps eliminate sore mouth,
  lips, and tongue

Helps fat, carbohydrate,
  and metabolism

Cancer prohibiting properties

**Deficiency Disease-**Ariboflavinosis (lip, mouth, skin, genitalia lesions)

### Signs of Deficiency

Cracks around mouth

Magenta color of tongue

Digestive disturbances

Anemia

Fatigue

Sluggishness

Scales on nose, face and
  ear lobes

Whiteheads on face and forehead

Broken blood vessel lines
  in cheek and nose

Oily skin

Burning sensation of hands
  and feet

Loss of hair

Baldness

Certain kinds of cataracts
  and blindness

Sensitivity to light

Frequent occurrence of bloodshot
  eyes

Dizziness

Trembling

Depression

Hysteria

Hypochondria

Inability to urinate

Vaginal itching

**Toxicity-**None known.

**Enemies-**Light, especially ultraviolet light and alkalines, water, sulfa, drugs, estrogen, alcohol, sugar.

**Natural Sources-**Brewer's yeast, milk, egg yolks, yogurt, whole grains, kidney, liver, heart and other organ meats, cheese, avocados, leafy vegetables, legumes, nuts, blackstrap molasses.

**Herb Sources-**Alfalfa, Blue Cohosh, Capsicum, Cascara, Catnip,

Chickweed, Dandelion, Eyebright, Fenugreek, Ginger, Goldenseal, Hawthorne, Hops, Kelp, Licorice, Marshmallow, Mullein, Papaya, Red Clover.

# VITAMIN B₃ (NIACIN OR NICOTINIC ACID, NIACINAMIDE)

**Water** soluble. Small quantities found in food usually need a supplement. Also called Vitamin P-P or Pellagra preventative. Called the happy vitamin because it helps with stress. A synthetic form of Niacin is used to enrich white flour products. Using amino acid tryptophan, the body can manufacture its own niacin.

## Positive Effects

Prevents Pellagra

Encourages optimism and happiness

Improves nervous system function

Being used to treat schizophrenics and autistic children

Migraine headache relief

Improves circulation of blood

Required for synthesis of sex hormones

Reduces complaints of cold hands and feet

Healthier looking skin

Helps proper function of skin and tongue

Helps proper function of digestive system

Helps metabolize proteins, fats, carbohydrates

Eases some cases of constipation and diarrhea

**Deficiency Disease-**Pellagra (depressing mental illness with insanity, delusion, violence, and death in later stages.)

## Signs of Deficiency

Depression

Suspicion

Unnecessary worry

Personality changes

Hostility

Loss of humor

Poor thinking

Poor memory

Mental dullness

Headaches

Hyperactive problems

Digestive problems

Halitosis

Backaches

**Toxicity-**Essentially non-toxic. Can cause flushing of the skin in some individuals. This will go away in 20-30 minutes. These individuals should decrease their dosage and make sure they take niacin with a B-Complex vitamin. Another form of Vitamin B3, niacinamide (also called nicotinamide), doesn't cause the flushing niacin (also called nicotinic acid) does. Niacin flushing can be minimized by taking it with a meal or with an equivalent amount of inositol. It is interesting to note that usually those who have a deficiency in this vitamin are the ones to have problems with flushing.

**Enemies-**Water, sulfa drugs, alcohol, food processing techniques, sleeping pills, estrogen, sugar.

**Natural Sources-**brewers yeast, liver, dessicated liver, turkey, tuna fish, chicken, lean meat, whole milk & milk products, rice bran, brown rice, peanuts, fish, whole cereals, dates, figs, prunes.

**Herb Sources-**Alfalfa, Blue Cohosh, Burdock, Capsicum, Catnip, Chickweed, Dandelion, Eyebright, Fenugreek, Ginger, Goldenseal, Hawthorne, Hops, Kelp, Licorice, Marshmallow, Mullein, Papaya, Red Clover, Rose Hips.

# VITAMIN B5 (PANTOTHENIC ACID, CALCIUM PANTOTHENATE, PANTHENOL)

Water soluble. Found in all living cells. Called anti-stress vitamin. Can be produced by natural occurring bacteria in the intestines. Major ingredient in honey bee's "royal jelly." Needed for PABA and Choline utilization.

NOTE: An investigation done in Japan has shown an interesting fact about Methyl Bromide and Pantothenic Acid. Methyl Bromide is an insecticidal fumigant that is used by food wholesalers to protect stored food from insects and rodents. It is used extensively in the United States and other countries because it leaves no odor, residue, or taste. It was found that food when sprayed with Methyl Bromide no longer contained any pantothenic acid. The pantothenic acid had been changed to a new, unknown element.

Another study done in England reported that today we only consume approximately one-fourth the thiamin (Vitamin B1) as peasants in England 500 years ago.

With these studies in mind, ask yourself: How many nutrients do we really get in our natural source? How good is your natural source? Are you overcooking or over-processing your food?

**Positive Effects**

Stress

Helps tingling hands and feet

Reduces adverse and toxic effects of many antibiotics

Addison's Disease

Prevents fatigue
Reduces Arthritis pain
**Taken with Calcium stops Bruxism (grinding of teeth at night)**
**Helps body withstand infection**
Builds antibodies
**Helps allergies and hay fever**
Wound healing
Used for post-operative shock

Helps metabolize fats, carbohydrates, and protein
Relieves flatulence
Intestinal tract paralysis
**Hypoglycemia**
**Hypoadrenia**
Stimulates adrenal hormonal production

**Deficiency Disease-**Hypoglycemia, blood and skin disorders, Hypoadrenia (adrenal exhaustion), Allergies.

**Signs of Deficiency-**Since all diseases are stress related and use extra anti-bodies, addition of extra pantothenic acid helps build body defenses.

Allergies
Hay fever
Respiratory problems
Skin disorders
Eczema
Furrowed tongue
Sore feet
Old age appearance
Malaise
Loss of hair
Gray hair
Abdominal pains
Flatulence
Vomiting
Diarrhea

Duodenal ulcers
Stomach ulcers
Headaches
Nerve problems
Neuritis
Loss of antibody production
Chronic sore throat
Anemia
Muscle cramps
Affects cellular health
Impairment of motor coordination
Kidney trouble
Sex gland trouble
Thyroid gland trouble

NOTE: There is some evidence that pantothenic acid stimulates the pituitary gland to put out natural cortisone. Cortisone is the hormone that helps control allergies. Also there is some evidence that arthritis may be caused by pantothenic acid deficiency.

**Toxicity-**None known.

**Enemies-**Heat, food processing techniques, canning, caffeine, sulfa drugs, sleeping pills, estrogen, alcohol, sugar.

**Natural Sources-**Egg yolks, kidneys, liver, milk, crude molasses, peanuts, brewers yeast, wheat germ, meat. Whole grains, bran, green vegetables, nuts, chicken, honey.
**Herb Sources-**Alfalfa, Black Cohosh, Blue Cohosh, Burdock, Capsicum, Cascara, Catnip, Chickweed, Dandelion, Eyebright, Fenugreek, Ginger, Goldenseal, Hawthorne, Hops, Horsetail, Kelp, Licorice, Marshmallow, Mullein, Papaya, Red Clover.

*Case History:*

F. suffered from chronic sore throat for over 30 years. She was given many different kinds of antibiotics, had her tonsils removed and even had cortisone shots in the nostril. She had tried using Vitamin A and C but it wasn't until she added 100 mg. of pantothenic acid every 3 or 4 hours that she saw any results. Then after 30 years of using drugs there was a remarkable change, she no longer had the chronic sore throat and hasn't for over 10 years.

# VITAMIN B6 (PYRIDOXINE)

Water soluble, it is excreted within eight hours of ingestion. Higher amounts are needed during pregnancy and lactation, and for people who smoke, use alcohol, or eat high protein diets. It is necessary for production of antibodies, DNA and RNA synthesis, red blood cells, and hydrochloric acid, and for magnesium assimilation. Helps metabolize fats, carbohydrates and protein; aids in absorption of B12; helps body fluid balance by regulating potassium and sodium levels in the body. Extra is needed if one is on the birth control pill. Vitamin B6 is excellent for controlling morning sickness. 200 mg. for 10 days and then 5 mg. thereafter to maintain has been used.

## Positive Effects

Controls nausea and vomiting in pregnancy
Natural diuretic-helps toxemia
Helps PMS (Premenstrual Syndrome)
Helps premenstrual anxiety, acne, and edema
Sexual disorders in men

Reduces hand numbness
Leg cramps
Helps muscular weakness
Prevention of rheumatism
Benefits people with atherosclerosis
Used in treatment of high cholesterol levels
Some heart disturbances

Helps hair loss
Helps acne, eczema, seborrhea
Stress
Helps insomnia
Helps Parkinson's Disease
Relieves convulsions in
  mentally retarded children
Neuritis in extremities
Reduces painful finger joints,
  burning feet
and heart attacks
Certain forms of diabetes
Anemia
Kidney stones
Ulcers
Hemorrhoids
Helps prevent tooth decay
Helps cancer immunity
Aids in conversion of tryptophan

## Deficiency Disease

Anemia, Seborrhic dermatitis, Glossitis, St. Vitus Dance.

## Signs of Deficiency

Nervousness
Irritability
Depression
Disturbance of good vision
Whiteheads on face, especially
  on forehead
Cracks in skin around eyes
  and mouth
Acne
Stretch marks (take with
  Zinc)
Hair loss
Immunity reduction
Morning sickness
Slow learning
Insomnia
Epilepsy
Edema during pregnancy
Premenstrual acne, edema,
  and anxieties
Muscular weakness
Staggering walk
Temporary paralysis of arm
  or leg
Arm and leg cramps
General weakness
Sensitivity to insulin
Unusual increased urination

**Toxicity-**None known.
**Enemies-**Long storage, canning, roasting, or stewing of meat, food processing techniques, alcohol, estrogen.
**Natural Sources-**Bananas, brewers yeast, beef, brown rice, cabbage, cantaloupe, carrots, black strap molasses, eggs, leafy, green vegetables, milk, organ meats, peanuts, wheat bran and germ.
**Herb Sources-**Alfalfa, Blue Cohosh, Burdock, Capsicum, Cascara, Catnip, Chickweed, Dandelion, Eyebright, Fenugreek, Ginger, Goldenseal, Hawthorne, Hops, Kelp, Licorice, Marshmallow, Mullein, Papaya, Red Clover.

# VITAMIN B₉ (FOLIC ACID OR FOLACIN)

Water soluble. Folic Acid was named because of the "foliage" in the plants that contain it. Also called the"other antianemia vitamin." Aids in the formation of red blood cells. It is needed for sugar and amino acid utilization, it helps the body to produce hydrochloric acid and helps to improve reproduction of new cells. It is important for the production of nucleic acids RNA and DNA. Some Folic Acid may be produced in the intestines. NOTE: There is a great need for Folic Acid during pregnancy to help prevent possible fetus damage and birth defects a Folic Acid deficiency could cause.

**Positive Effects**

Forestalls greying hair
Prevents canker sores
Helps menstrual difficulties
Helps prevent pregnancy
    complications including:
    cleft palate, slow development
    potential, brain damage,
    premature delivery, afterbirth
    hemorrhaging and early
    placenta separation
Improves lactation
Wards off anemia
Increases intelligence

Treats dropsy, diarrhea
    and leg ulcers
Helps atherosclerosis and
    gout
Synthesis of DNA and RNA
Helps building and repairing
    of body
Decreases disease susceptibility
Helps prevent some intestinal
    parasites
Helps prevent food poisoning
Increases appetite if debilitated

**Deficiency Disease-**Megaloblastic Anemia, Nutritional Macrocytic Anemia, Pernicious Anemia.

**Signs of Deficiency-**Folic Acid deficiency is not uncommon. Two groups are especially susceptible—pregnant women, because of the extra demands for folic acid from the fetus, and people suffering from injury or severe illness, because of the demands to repair their bodies.

Tongue inflammation
Cankers
Gastrointestinal troubles
Greying hair
Increased disease susceptibility
Easily fatigued
Weak

Irritability
Sleeplessness
Forgetfulness
Mental derangement
Schizophrenic delusions
Withdrawal
Catatonia

**Toxicity-**None known.

**Enemies-**Heat, light, long unprotected storage at room temperature, water, sulfa drugs, estrogen, food processing-especially boiling.

**Natural Sources-**Dark, leafy green vegetables (Broccoli, spinach, etc.), peanuts, beans, organ meats, brewers yeast, root vegetables, egg yolk, cantaloupe, apricots, parsley, avocados, whole wheat, dark rye flour.

**Herb Sources-**Alfalfa, Blue Cohosh, Burdock, Capsicum, Cascara, Catnip, Chickweed, Dandelion, Eyebright, Fenugreek, Ginger, Goldenseal, Hawthorne, Hops, Kelp, Licorice, Marshmallow, Mullein, Papaya, Red Clover.

# VITAMIN B$_{12}$ (COBALAMIN)

Water soluble. Called the red vitamin. Unlike most water soluble vitamins it can be stored by the body. It is necessary for proper carbohydrate, fat and protein metabolism. It is necessary for the body's use of some amino acids and Vitamin D. It assists in the development of red blood cells and aids the body in the utilization of iron. A greater need for B$_{12}$ exists during pregnancy.

People who are deficient in B$_{12}$ develop Pernicious Anemia. (Folic Acid also helps B$_{12}$ to prevent Pernicious Anemia) Many times B12 is injected rather than given orally when a deficiency is suspected because of the inability of a deficient body to absorb it. B$_{12}$ needs to be combined with Calcium.

**Positive Effects**

| | |
|---|---|
| Healthy nervous system | Relieves loss of ability |
| Relief of nervousness | to concentrate |
| Relief of memory loss | Improves mental state |
| Relieves irritability | Prevents anemia |
| Relieves insomnia | Helps bronchial asthma |
| Treats depression and fatigue | Helps growth |
| Relief of loss of balance | Helps some skin problems |
| Improves coordination | Possible anti-viral action |
| Increase energy | Greater resistance to germs |

**Deficiency Disease-**Pernicious Anemia, Brain Damage. (Permanent mental and physical damage if deficiency is extreme even paralysis if not corrected.)

**Signs of Deficiency-**Subtle changes in the nervous system with the following four signs occurring together. 1. Reduced sensory perception, 2. Jerky motion of the limbs, 3. Weakness of arms and legs, 4. Trouble walking and speaking.

Schizophrenia-like mental disorders or associated brain damage

Nervousness and irritability

Tingling or burning sensations of hands and feet.

Pale, white lipped

Ringing in ears

Spots before eyes

Abdominal difficulties- gas, constipation or diarrhea, nausea, vomiting, pain, poor appetite.

Unpleasant body odors

Menstrual problems

Dandruff

Heart palpitations

Sore tongue

**Toxicity-**None known even with large amounts given.

**Enemies-**Acids, alkalies, water, sunlight, alcohol, estrogen, sleeping pills.

**Natural Sources-**Because Animal protein is almost the only natural source of adequate amounts of B 12 people on vegetarian diets are advised to take supplements.

Liver, kidney, cheese, eggs, milk, fish, sunflower seeds, organ meats, raw wheat germ, pollen, beef, lamb.

**Herb Sources-**Alfalfa, Bee Pollen, Blue Cohosh, Burdock, Capsicum, Cascara, Catnip, Chickweed, Dandelion, Dong Quai, Eyebright, Fenugreek, Ginger, Ginseng, Goldenseal, Hawthorne, Hops, Kelp, Licorice, Marshmallow, Mullein, Papaya, Red Clover, White Oak Bark.

# VITAMIN B₁₅ (PANGAMIC ACID)

Pangamic Acid is a water soluble vitamin used extensively in Russia. In the United States, the Food and Drug Administration (FDA) wants it off the market. Hopefully given time Pangamic Acid will have the chance to prove itself.

Pangamic Acid is an example of why not to depend upon vitamin supplements as the only way to obtain your needed nutrients. Man can only put in a pill what he is allowed to by government restrictions and by what knowledge he has. Some vitamins are still undiscovered. Nature has these nutrients in the herbs and plants she provides for us. Supplements should be just that—a supplement, not a diet.

**Positive Effects**

Extend cell life span

Helps fatigue

Protects against pollutants

Protects the liver against cirrhosis

Lower blood cholesterol levels

| Aids protein synthesis | Relieve symptoms of angina |
|---|---|
| Stops the craving for liquor | and asthma |
| Ward off hangovers | Stimulate immunity responses |

**Deficiency Disease-**see below

**Signs of Deficiency-**There is limited research but indications are glandular and nerve disorders, heart disease and diminished oxygenation of living tissue.

**Toxicity-**none. Some experience nausea when beginning to take B 15.

**Enemies-**Water and sunlight.

**Herb Sources-**Black Walnut.

# VITAMIN B₁₇ (LAETRILE)

Laetrile is an extremely controversial vitamin. It is available in the United States on a limited basis for cancer research.

Laetrile contains natural cyanide and has been used to kill cancer cells. Normal cells contain a substance called rhodanese that cancer cells lack. When the cyanide from laetrile comes in contact with a normal cell, rhodanese neutralizes or detoxifies it. When the cyanide comes in contact with a cancer cell, it kills it because it has no rhodanese to protect it. One side says laetrile is a selective cancer killer that only targets cancer cells and leaves normal cells unharmed. The other side says laetrile contains a substance-cyanide that is poisonous and harmful to the body. Each side is vocal and sure they are right.

The author makes no recommendation either for or against laetrile. This information (as is all information in this book) is presented only as that—information. It is your responsibility to study and make your own decision.

**Positive Effects-**Those in favor of laetrile say it is a cancer preventative and cure. That it will decrease the size of malignant tumors, ease their pain and suppress the growth of cancerous tissue.

**Deficiency Disease-**unknown.

**Signs of Deficiency-**Those in favor of laetrile say a reduced resistance to cancer will occur if one is deficient.

**Toxicity-**none established. Those against laetrile warn care and caution because of the cyanide. We would warn against some unethical people who promise "everything."

**Natural Sources-**Pits of apricots, peaches, apples, cherries, nectarines, and plums. Some who wish to take laetrile for the possible benefits eat a few apple seeds when they eat an apple. To them this small amount seems prudent.

# VITAMIN C (ASCORBIC ACID)

Water soluble. The first vitamin discovered by man when a cure for scurvy was found. Needs to be replaced daily. It is best taken after or with a meal or snack. Most animals manufacture their own Vitamin C but man, apes and guinea pigs are among the few who do not.

An antioxidant and a universal antitoxin, which means it helps protect against harmful oxidation that damages cells and protects against poisonous and harmful substances of all kinds. It has a primary role in the formation of collagen and helps the body's absorption of iron.

1000 mg. of Vitamin C taken every hour at the first sign of a cold or illness has been very effective for some people. This amount is continued until the symptoms leave. If Vitamin C is taken in mega-doses for more than 3 or 4 days, it can act as a chelating agent and flush out Vitamin B and Calcium from the body. Taking extra B Complex and Calcium when you use these higher doses of C prevents this.

Some feel the need for Vitamin C is over-rated. However, the U.S. Department of Agriculture found Vitamin C one of four nutrients most wanting in the American diet.

**Positive Effects**

Wards off disease
Fights bacterial and viral
    infections
Prevents Scurvy
Prevents and treats Hepatitis
Polio
Diabetes
Cancer
Helps with cataracts and
    eye infections
Helps those with back complaints
Allergies and sinus problems
Useful in ulcer treatment
Gallstones
Adrenal Glands
Prickly Heat

Tonsil and ear infections
Common cold
Childhood diseases
Helps prevent high blood
    cholesterol
Helps prevent arteriosclerosis
    and atherosclerosis

Helps walls of blood vessels
Improves circulation and
    blood
Frostbite and freezing pre-
    ventative
Energy
Protects against oxidants
Detoxifies many common drugs

May act as preventative
for crib death
Acts as a natural laxative
Can substitute for other
water soluble vitamins lacking
in the body.
Used heavily during stress
Helps the body handle stress
Useful in treating schizophrenia
Increases mental ability
Builds teeth, prevents caries
Prevents pyorrhea
Lowers incidence of blood
clots in the veins
Ease joint movement
Extend life by helping
protein cells to hold together

Detoxifies insect bites,
poison ivy, and oak
Neutralizes poisoning-
mercury, carbon monoxide,
arsenic, benzene, bromides,
nitrites, cadmium, air
pollution, severe overdoses
of aspirin, etc.
Youthful looks
Helps complexion
Helps fingernails
Hastens and aids the healing
process of wounds, injuries
and burns.
Maintains healthy connective
tissue (skin and ligaments)
Helps with arthritis

**Deficiency Disease-** Scurvey. Some researchers believe Atherosclerosis is a deficiency disease of Vitamin C.

**Signs of Deficiency**

Poor digestion and appetite
Permanent goose bumps
Anemia
Susceptibility to disease
Swollen and painful joints
Bleeding gums
Nosebleeds
Easy bruising
Poor lactation

Bone and teeth weakness
General Debility
High cholesterol levels
Rheumatism
Intestinal trouble
Irritability
Softening of the bones
Fatigue

**Toxicity-**none.

**Enemies-**Stress, smoking, high fever, aspirin, pain killers, water, cooking, heat, light, oxygen, alcohol.

**Natural Source-**fresh fruits, (apples) fresh vegetables (potatoes, broccoli, cabbage), acerola cherries, tomatoes, rose hips, green or red peppers.

**Herb Sources-**Alfalfa, Barberry, Bayberry, Bee Pollen, Burdock, Capsicum, Catnip, Chickweed, Comfrey, Dandelion, Echinacea, Eyebright, Fennel, Garlic, Ginger, Goldenseal, Hawthorne, Juniper, Kelp, Papaya, Parsley, Peppermint, Pole Root, Red Clover, Thyme, Yarrow, Yellow Dock.

# VITAMIN D (CALCIFEROL, VIOSTEROL, ERGOS-TEROL)

Fat soluble. Body stores it, particularly in the liver. It is critical for bone and teeth development. It has been called the "**nerve**" vitamin because it helps the body assimilate calcium.

Also called the "**Sunshine vitamin**" because it is manufactured by the body when the ultraviolet rays of the sun act on the oils of the skin. The body then absorbs it from the skin. (Note: When vitamin D is taken orally it is absorbed with fats through the intestinal wall.) Lighter skin allows greater amounts of Vitamin D to be produced and darker skin inhibits it. Our bodies have a built-in safety factor of suntanning. in fact some researchers believe that sunstroke may be related to excessive intake of Vitamin D. With caution and gradual exposure to the sun (morning sun is best) we stay in the guidelines the Lord intended for our bodies.

Smog blocks the sun's rays from getting to the skin. People in heavy polluted areas should be aware of their Vitamin D needs.

## Positive Effects

Helps body absorb calcium
and phosphorus
Aids sleep and nerves relax
because of calcium absorption
Increases bone density
Important to bone (and teeth)
growth, development and
health
Helps bone loss
Helps mending of broken
bones
Helps make straight legs

Prevents tooth decay
Prevents acids in mouth
from harming teeth
Strong, white teeth
Helps development of face
Helps skin health
Helps myopia
Aids Vitamin A assimilation
Prevents colds (take with
A and C)
Helps treat conjunctivitis
Helps rheumatoid arthritis

**Deficiency Disease**-Rickets, Osteomalacia, Tetany, Severe tooth decay, Senile osteoporosis.
## Signs of Deficiency

Rickets-bowed legs, funnel
chest, other bone deformities
Osteomalacia-softening
of bones
Tetany-muscle spasms, numbness
with sensations of tingling

Cramps
Diarrhea
Dementia
Dermatitis
Insanity
Nervousness

Severe tooth decay
Senile Osteoporosis-porous
   and fragile, brittle bones
Muscular and nervous weaknesses
Constipation
Gas

Insomnia
Pellagra
Sunburned appearance
Rough scaly skin
Burning sensations in mouth
   and throat

**Toxicity-**It is considered possible to overdose Vitamin D because it is a fat soluble vitamin. 30,000 I.U. daily for infants, 50,000 I.U. daily for children, and 100,000-150,000 I.U. daily for adults can be toxic **if taken over an extended period of time.**

Note: The cases of hypervitaminosis (overdosage) of Vitamin D that have brought on this scare of toxicity were when the synthetic Vitamin D was used. Do not take synthetic vitamins especially in large doses. We do not feel that natural Vitamin D is toxic; however taking massive doses of any fat soluble vitamin (except Vitamin E) is not advocated unless a severe deficiency is present.

**Enemies-**Smog, mineral oil

**Natural Sources-**Fish liver oils, salmon, herring, sardines, tuna, egg yolks, bone meal, organ meats.

**Herb Sources-**Alfalfa, Bee Pollen, Chickweed, Eyebright, Fenugreek, Mullein, Papaya, Red Raspberry, Rosehips, Sarsaparilla.

# VITAMIN E (TOCOPHEROL)

Fat soluble. Unlike other fat soluble vitamins it is stored for a short period of time in the body and then any extra is eliminated in the feces. The word tocopherol is Greek for "ability to bear young." Vitamin E's reputation for helping fertility is well known.

Taking Selenium with E increases the power of E. Manganese needs to be present in the body for vitamin E to be effective.

Vitamin E is an antioxidant. The oxidation of body cells is the partial cause of aging. Vitamin E has been used to retard aging. (Synthetic E will not prevent the oxidation of Vitamin A.) It also helps cell respiration so cells are able to manage with less oxygen.

The blood flow is improved by Vitamin E and it causes blood vessels to dilate or expand. It is an inhibitor of improper blood coagulation thus it helps prevent blood clots. It has been called nature's blood thinner. However, unlike chemical blood thinners it does not cause hemorrhaging. I have used a poked capsule of E many times to stop bleeding in the mouth.

Books have been written on Vitamin E, along with Vitamin C. There is probably more research on them than any other vitamin. It is impossible to list *all* the information even in condensed form. Let's summarize by saying this section offers you a taste of what Vitamin E is capable of doing. It seems to be the "everything" vitamin for "everything."

**Positive Effects**

Speeds wound healing
Prevents internal and external
 scar tissue
Accelerates healing of burns
Reduces aging process
Removes and prevents wrinkles
Removes liver spots (100
 mg. after each meal for
 6 weeks)
Increases fertility
Restores potency in men
Prevents miscarriage
Prevents muscular dystrophy
 in children when taken by
 pregnant women.
Helps pain of varicose veins
Aids menstrual problems
Holds off menopause
Helps disorders of menopause
Dissolves and prevents blood
 clots
Used for heart disease, especially
 coronary thrombosis

Improves circulation
Heart failure repair and
 prevention
Lowers cholesterol levels,
 take with Vitamin A
Enhances activity of A
Works as a diuretic, can
 lower blood pressure
Relieves pain in arms and
 legs
Alleviates fatigue
Necessary for proper muscle
 functioning
Helps muscle tone and strength
Protects lungs against air
 pollution
Relief of migraine headaches
Visual problems, crossed
 eyes, and nearsightedness
May retard cancer
Effective in large doses
 for muscular dystrophy
Stops cold sores

**Deficiency Disease -**Reproductive disorder, muscle degeneration, destruction of red blood cells, anemia.

**Signs of Deficiency**

Reproductive failure, dis-
 orders, miscarriages
Fertility problems
Loss of sexual interest
Stillbirths
Anemia and edema
 in premature babies
 and undernourished infants

Dull, falling hair
Heart problems
Coronary thrombosis
Nephritis
Improper blood clotting
Skin problems
Muscular weaknesses

**Toxicity-**none. Some precautions are suggested for High Blood Pressure and Rheumatic heart cases. While Vitamin E is used to help both of these problems initial doses should be small and monitored to give the heart and circulatory system time to adjust to the improved efficiency that Vitamin E gives. Vitamin E works to lower blood pressure but it may first raise it. For Rheumatic heart cases initial doses of 90 I.U. a day for another month and increased to 150 I.U. a day for the rest of the time with no further increase. Rheumatic heart cases seem to do best on the smaller doses.

Note: Watching for results can sometimes be amazing because it works so quickly for some conditions, and frustrating because for other conditions (especially chronic conditions) it works as a slow gradual process often seemingly without results for weeks or months.

**Enemies-**Heat, oxygen, freezing temperatures, food processing, inorganic iron, chlorine, mineral oil, frying.

**Natural Sources-**Cold pressed vegetable oils- safflower, sunflower, soybean, whole wheat, whole grain cereals, nuts, grain, molasses, organ meats, eggs, sweet potatoes, broccoli, brussel sprouts, leafy greens, spinach.

**Herb Sources-**Alfalfa, Bee Pollen, Blue Cohosh, Burdock, Comfrey, Dandelion, Dong Quai, Echinecea, Eyebright, Ginseng, Goldenseal, Kelp, Licorice, Papaya, Red Raspberry, Rose Hips, Skullcap, Slippery Elm, Yarrow.

# VITAMIN F (LINOLEIC ACID, LINOLENIC ACID, ARACHADONIC ACID)

Consists of unsaturated fatty acids. Some writers call them Vitamin F, others call them essential fatty acids—meaning they are essential for good health. However, the body's need and use of them is very similar to its use of other vitamins.

The body is unable to make unsaturated fatty acids. However, if there is sufficient linoleic acid present the other two fatty acids can be synthesized. These unsaturated fats help burn saturated fat in the body, thus they play a major role in preventing and alleviating cholestrol build-up.

One of the most important functions of Vitamin F is in helping gland function, particularly the adrenals and the thyroid.

Fatty acids are stored in the fat tissues of the body. Having sufficient Vitamin F can help weight loss, but an excess can lead to unwanted pounds. We need enough but not too much. An excellent way to obtain these nutrients is to use cold pressed oils in our diet (See natural sources). If taken as a supplement it is best taken with meals.

**Positive Effects**

Aids oxygen through blood stream

Assists respiration of body organs

Aids cellular health

Helps proper nourishment of skin

Lubricates body cells

Regulates coagulation of blood

Healthy mucous membranes

Doesn't increase body's need for Vitamin E as does saturated fats

Helps nerves to be healthy

Helps reproductive system function properly

Healthy skin, hair

Helps glands, especially thyroid and adrenals

Aids in weight reduction

Aids in growth, well-being

Treats acne, eczema

Combats heart disease

Some protection against harmful effects of X-rays

**Deficiency Disease-**Eczema, Acne
**Signs of Deficiency**

Cholesterol Buildup

Acne

Dry Skin

Eczema

Dry, brittle, dull hair

Dandruff

Diarrhea

Gallstones

Underweight

Varicose Veins

Swelling of edema

Loss of sex drive

Decline of friendly bacteria

**Toxicity-**none—excess can lead to unwanted pounds.
**Enemies-**Saturated Fats, heat, oxygen
**Natural Sources-**safflower oil, sunflower oil and seeds, corn oil, soybean oil, peanut oil, wheat germ, peanuts, walnuts, pecans, almonds, avocados, cottonseed oil, (not Brazil nuts and cashews)
**Herb Sources-**Red Raspberry, Silppery Elm, Yarrow.

# VITAMIN H--BIOTIN (COENZYME R)

Water soluble, B complex family member. It is found in small amounts in all living tissue. It can be synthesized by the intestinal bacteria. It is essential to the metabolism of carbohydrates, proteins, fat and unsaturated fatty acids. A substance in raw egg whites called avidin prevents absorption of biotin. If raw eggs are eaten extra biotin is necessary. Also balding men, pregnant or nursing women, those on antibiotics or sulfa drugs should consider their extra biotin needs.

Some skin diseases (Seborrhea, Dermatitis) in infants have been linked to biotin deficiencies. It is interesting to note that breast milk contains biotin.

## Positive Effects

Necessary for metabolism of carbohydrates, protein, fats, especially unsaturated fatty acids.

Normal growth

Maintains healthy skin, sebaceous glands, nerves, and bone marrow.

Helps proper functions of sex glands

Promotes mental health

Eases muscle pains

Used to treat hair loss and baldness

Healthy hair

Aids in keeping hair from turning gray

Alleviates eczema, seborrhea, dermatitis

**Deficiency Disease-**Eczema of face and body, Extreme exhaustion, Impairment of fat metabolism, Heart conditions, Paralysis, Infant Skin Diseases.

## Signs of Deficiency

Dermatitis

Dry, peeling skin

Skin infection

Mouth and lip sores

Pallor

Poor appetite

Nausea and vomiting

Stunted growth

Pains around heart

Cancers expand rapidly

Muscle pains

Lack of energy

Sleeplessness

Extreme fatigue

Hair falling out

Mental depression

Nervous system disturbances

Heart troubles

Tickling sensations of hands and feet

**Toxicity-**none known.

**Enemies-**Raw egg whites, sulfa drugs, antibiotics, estrogen, food-processing techniques, alcohol.

**Natural Sources-**Brewers yeast, egg yolks, kidney, liver, wheat germ, rolled oats, nuts, chicken, lamb, brown rice, beans, nuts, peanuts, beef, veal, fish, cheese, milk.

**Herb Sources-**Alfalfa, Blue Cohosh, Burdock, Capsicum, Cascara, Catnip, Chickweed, Dandelion, Eyebright, Fenugreek, Ginger, Goldenseal, Hawthorne, Hops, Kelp, Licorice, Marshmallow, Mullein, Papaya, Red Clover.

## VITAMIN K (MENADINE)

Was named for the Danish word for blood clotting-*Koagulation.* It is important in the production of the clotting agent prothrombin and in the conversion of glucose to glycogen (the form of sugar stored in the body for use as fuel.)

Vitamin K is produced in the intestines of normal, healthy people. It is important for normal function of the liver and needs bile to be utilized.

**Positive Effects**

Promotes proper blood clotting

Reduces hemorrhaging

Used in treatment of coronary thrombosis

Used to prepare women for childbirth

Aids in reducing excessive menstrual flow

**Deficiency Disease-**Colitis, Celiac disease, Nutrient absorption difficulties in intestines, Improper blood clotting, Sprue.

**Signs of Deficiency**

Improper blood clotting

Internal bleeding or hemorrhages

Bleeding from bladder, intestines

Bleeding from mouth, nose

Nutrient absorption diseases

Colitis

Excessive diarrhea

**Toxicity-**Natural Vitamin K is nontoxic. Synthetic Vitamin K can be toxic and can produce some forms of anemia or cause damage to the red blood cells of infants. Toxic effects include: chest constriction, sweating and flushing of skin. Supplements of Vitamin K are usually not available. It is best to get it from food.

**Natural Sources-**fish liver oils, kelp, soybeans and oil, safflower oil, egg yolks, alfalfa, leafy green vegetables, spinach, tomatoes, potatoes, yogurt, corn, strawberries, wheat bran and germ, cauliflower, carrots, peas, cow's milk. Main source for humans is from intestinal flora manufacturing it.

**Herb Sources-**Alfalfa, Gotu Kola,Papaya, Safflower, Slippery Elm, Yarrow.

# VITAMIN P (BIOFLAVONOIDS)

Called Vitamin P after paprika, the spice from which it was first isolated. Water soluble. Actually a bioflavonoid complex consisting of rutin, hesperidin and citrin. Found in the pulp of fruits and vegetables. The best way to get bioflavonoids is to eat fruit with the peel or leave some of the white pulp in citrus fruits on the fruit.

Aids the functions of Vitamin C in keeping collagen (connective tissue of cells) healthy. It also aids the action of the capillaries in allowing nutrients in and body wastes out. Bioflavonoids are called the **capillary permeability factor**. It controls the size of the tiny holes in the capillaries, keeping them large enough to allow nutrients through; but too small for viruses, that may cause disease, or blood cells, that could lead to hemorrhaging, to pass through.

**Positive Effects-**(See also Vitamin C)

Works synergistically with
    Vitamin C
Prevents bruising
Strengthens capillary walls
Protects against excessive
    blood clotting
Protects against arterial
    degeneration
Builds resistance to disease
Relieves menopausal hot flashes
    when taken with Vitamin C

Prevents, heals bleeding
    gums
Prevents Vitamin C from
    being oxidized
Treatment of ulcers
Treatment of asthma
Treatment of edema (natural
    diuretic)
Treatment of dizziness due
    to inner ear problems

**Deficiency Disease-**Capillary fragility
**Signs of Deficiency-**(See Vitamin C)

Easy bruising and bleeding
Nose bleeds
Bleeding gums
Heavy menstrual bleeding
Habitual threatened miscarriage

Postpartum bleeding
Skin disorders
Diabetes retinitis
Hemorrhoids
Edema

**Toxicity-**non-toxic

**Enemies-**boiling, air, water, cooking, heat, light, smoking.
**Natural Sources-**White skin and pulp of oranges, lemons, and grapefruit, apricots, cherries, grapes, plums, papaya, prunes, cantaloupe, blackberries, paprika, and red pepper (cayenne) buckwheat, rosehips, tomatoes, broccoli, spinach.
**Herb Sources-**Burdock, Dandelion, Red Clover, Rose Hips, Slippery Elm, Cayenne.

# VITAMIN U

Many people do not recognize this vitamin exists. Very little is known about Vitamin U. It is used for treating ulcers. Fresh cabbage juice regimes have effectively healed stomach ulcers in as little as 11 days.
**Positive Effects-**important role in healing ulcers, duodenal and peptic.
**Toxicity-**none known.
**Enemies-**heat
**Natural Sources-**Raw cabbage, raw cabbage juice, homemade sauerkraut, celery, raw celery juice, fresh greens, raw egg yolks, raw milk.
**Herb Sources-**Alfalfa.

# CHOLINE

Not "officially" recognized as a vitamin. It is a member of the B-Complex family. Choline is a component of lecithin. It is a fat emulsifier and works with Inositol, another B-complex vitamin, to dissolve and utilize fats and cholesterol. It can be made by the body. It goes directly to the brain to help produce lecithin, which contains choline. Cow's milk does not contain lecithin.
**Positive Effects**

| | |
|---|---|
| Aids utilization of fats and cholesterol | Aids and improves memory |
| | Helps conquer memory loss |
| Helps prevent coronary thrombosis and coronary occlusion | Soothing effect on body |
| | Maintains a healthy liver |
| Helps arteriosclerosis | Viral hepatitis |
| Helps leg cramps caused from blockage in circulation | Helps liver eliminate poisons and drugs from the system |
| Helps high blood pressure | Aids function of gall bladder |
| Used to treat glaucoma | Aids the thymus, spleen |

| | |
|---|---|
| Helps kidney disease | Inhibits cancer growth in |
| Aids diabetes | animals |
| Aids Muscular Dystrophy | Aids myelin sheath |

**Deficiency Disease-**Cirrhosis and fatty degeneration of the liver, hardening of the arteries, and possibly Alzheimer's Disease.

**Signs of Deficiency-**

| | |
|---|---|
| Liver problems | Vision difficulties |
| Hardening of arteries | Nervousness or twitching |
| High blood pressure | Growth problems |
| Bleeding stomach ulcers | Dizziness |
| Kidney hemorrhage | Noises in the ear |
| Kidney tube blockage | Sleeplessness |

**Toxicity-**None known, too much may lead to a deficiency in Vitamin B6.

**Enemies-**Water, sulfa drugs, estrogen, food processing, alcohol.

**Natural Sources-**Wheat germ, egg yolks, fish, liver, desiccated liver, organ meats, brewers yeast, lecithin, soybeans, green leafy vegetables, peanuts.

**Herb Sources-**Alfalfa, Blue Cohosh, Burdock, Capsicum, Cascara, Catnip, Chickweed, Dandelion, Eyebright, Fenugreek, Ginger, Goldenseal, Hawthorne, Hops, Kelp, Licorice, Marshmallow, Mullein, Papaya, Red Clover.

# INOSITOL

Water soluble. Part of the B Complex family. It combines with choline to form lecithin. It is one of those vitamins not recognized as essential to human health by the Food and Nutrition Board, however, the body doesn't seem to agree with the board. The human body in its normal state contains more inositol than any other vitamin except for Niacin (Vitamin B3.)

It is abundant in heart muscle and occurs in extraordinarily high concentrations in the human brain. It has been called **a brain nourisher.**

Heavy coffee drinkers, alcohol consumers, and women after menopause need extra Inositol.

**Positive Effects**

| | |
|---|---|
| Aids brain nutrition | Prevents hardening of arteries |
| Necessary to brain activity | Helps arteriosclerosis |
| Vitamin E utilization | Lowers and controls cholesterol levels |

Synergistic with E in treating
nerve damage
Cerebral Palsy
Multiple dystrophy
Nerves
Retarded mentality
Aids body in fat metabolism
Breaks up and aids in body
fat distribution
Prevents circulatory ailments
Important to hair growth
Prevents baldness
Necessary to Eye function

Corrects heart muscle function
Protects kidneys, liver
and heart.
Necessary to the action
of the liver
Prevents fatty liver
Helps gall bladder trouble
Helps diabetes
Prevents eczema
Helps crossed eyes and eye
abnormalities

**Deficiency Disease-**Eczema
**Signs of Deficiency-**
Skin problems
Eczema
Eye abnormalities
Eye trouble

High blood cholesterol
Constipation
Hair loss

A deficiency may be caused by large doses of caffeine.
**Toxicity-**none.
**Enemies-**Caffeine, coffee, water, sulfa drugs, estrogen, food poisoning, alcohol.
**Natural Sources-**Lecithin, brewers yeast, wheat germ, beef brains and heart, organ meats, liver, blackstrap molasses, citrus fruits, cereals, dried beans, cantaloupe, raisins, brown rice, peanuts, nuts, cabbage, oatmeal, whole wheat bread, milk.
**Herb Sources-**Alfalfa, Blue Cohosh, Burdock, Capsicum, Cascara, Catnip, Chickweed, Dandelion, Eyebright, Fenugreek, Ginger, Goldenseal, Hawthorne, Hops, Kelp, Licorice, Marshmallow, Mullein, Papaya, Red Clover.

# PABA (PARA-AMINO BENZOIC ACID)

Water soluble. B complex family. It is actually a "vitamin within a vitamin" since it is one of the basic parts of folic acid. It helps with production of folic acid in the intestines. If conditions are right PABA can be synthesized in the intestines.

It aids in the metabolism of protein, helps in the assimilation of pantothenic acid, and has been used in suntan preparation because it acts as a sunscreen.

PABA is antagonistic to sulfa drugs. Sulfa drugs combine with the same things that PABA does so the one that is in greater quantity crowds the other one out. PABA can make sulfa drugs ineffective and sulfa drugs can cause a PABA deficiency as well deficiencies of folic acid and pantothenic acid.

**Positive Effects-**

Maintains health of intestines

Helps protein metabolism

Helps folic acid production

Pantothenic acid assimilation

Has sunscreen properties

Protects against skin cancer from overexposure to the skin

Helps a woman to conceive

Used as treatment for vitiligo

Reduces pain of burns

Important to skin health

Used with folic acid to restore natural haircolor

Delays effects of aging on skin, wrinkles, dark spots, etc.

**Deficiency Disease-**Eczema

**Signs of Deficiency**

Digestive disorders

Fatigue

Depression

Nervousness

Irritability

Hallucinations

**Toxicity-**none known. However, large doses for long periods of time are not recommended.

**Enemies-**Sulfa drugs, water, food-processing techniques, alcohol, estrogen.

**Natural Sources-**Brewers yeast, wheat germ, whole grains, bran, rice, molasses, liver, kidney, milk, eggs, yogurt.

**Herb Sources-**Alfalfa, Blue Cohosh, Burdock, Capsicum, Cascara, Catnip, Chickweed, Dandelion, Eyebright, Fenugreek, Ginger, Goldenseal, Hawthorne, Hops, Horsetail, Kelp, Licorice, Marshmallow, Mullein, Papaya, Red Clover.

# MINERALS

Minerals are similar to vitamins in many ways; they are necessary for basic life processes and for good health. Minerals act as catalysts throughout the body. They are necessary to activate many vitamins. Animals and plants must obtain them from an outside source. Plants extract them from the soil and animals get minerals from plants. One reason herbs benefit the body so much is because of their high mineral content, including trace minerals.

A difference between vitamins and minerals is that vitamins are "used up" by the body whereas minerals stay the same and make up actual structures in the body. Calcium and phosphorus in the bones are good examples of this. We need a fresh supply of minerals because there is a constant mineral turnover.

Many times vitamins and minerals work together; a good example is calcium and vitamin D. Shortage of minerals may also result in deficiency diseases such as rickets (Calcium and Vitamin D), goiter (Iodine), anemia (Iron) and others. Lesser deficiencies give rise to tension, insomnia, fatigue, depression, irritability, skin and hair problems, etc.

## Chelated Minerals

Chelation-(pronounced key- lation) a process of wrapping the mineral in a molecule of protein. (Hydrolized protein or amino acids are commonly used.) This is essential since the blood stream will not accept a mineral until it has been chelated. If the mineral is not accepted by the body to activate vitamins, then both the vitamin and mineral will pass from the system with no benefit. The body must chelate minerals itself before they can be used.

The first thing the body must do to chelate a mineral is dissolve it. After the body dissolves the mineral, it uses protein to chelate the mineral. Then the body can accept the mineral. Very often the body is unable to dissolve these hard minerals either because of poor digestion or because of taking a mineral in a form the body cannot use. There is evidence that taking minerals in a pre-chelated form makes sure the body can use them. Taking supplements with meals or with digestive enzyme supplements is another way to help assimilation because of the protein, enzymes, etc., in the food.

# CALCIUM

Warm milk at bedtime is a popular grandmother's remedy for sleep problems. Perhaps a good calcium supplement would be better because it wouldn't cause the mucus-forming problems of milk; but grandma certainly had the right idea. Calcium acts as a natural tranquilizer and sleep aid.

There is more calcium, an essential mineral, in the body than any other mineral. Almost all of it is in the bones and teeth. Calcium is not "used up" like vitamins. It makes up the actual structure of the bones and teeth. Approximately 20% of adult bone calcium is reabsorbed and replaced every year.

**Facts about Calcium**
— aids in metabolism and is essential to the muscles.
— must have sufficient Vitamin D to absorb it.
— Calcium loss is retarded by exercise.
— Calcium absorption goes down in the elderly.
— Emotional stress can flush Calcium out of the system at a higher rate.
— Works with Phosphorus in a 2 to 1 relationship for bone and teeth health.
— Calcium and iron are the 2 most deficient minerals in the American women's diet.
— Included in the Department of Agriculture's list of 4 most missing nutrients.—*People who require extra calcium:* pregnant and lactating women, infants and growing children, the elderly, hypoglycemics, and those who have backaches, menstrual cramps, growing pains, leg aches or charlie horses.

**Positive Effects**

Nerve function-impulse transmission
Natural tranquilizer
Alleviates insomnia
Nerves-stress
Helps premenstrual syndrome
Helps headache pain
Excellent pain killer (1-4 grams of Calcium and a Vitamin D pill has been used for dental pain)
Calcium injections have been used for pleurisy,

Leg cramps
Charlie horses
Strong bones and teeth
Treats rickets
Treats Arthritis
Treats osteoporosis
Works with magnesium for cardiovascular health
Helps regulate the heart beat
Lowers cholesterol and triglycerides
Helps proper blood clotting

migraine, broken ribs,
labor pains, arthritis,
muscle aches and cramps,
menopausal disorders,
& allergic reactions.
Muscle contractions

Iron metabolism
Helps Vitamin C functions
Helps prevent skin trouble
Large amounts may help alleviate
    some signs of aging

**Deficiency Disease-**Rickets, Osteomalacia, Osteoporosis
(See Vitamin D)

**Signs of Deficiency**

Poor growth
Growing pains
Muscle and nerve irritability
Teeth decaying
Gum inflammation (periodontal
    disease)
Heart palpitations
Fragile bones
Muscle cramps

Weak muscles
Painful joints
Arthritis
Backaches
Menstrual cramps
Cataracts
Paralysis
Multiple sclerosis
Sleep problems

**Toxicity-**Divided theories—most researchers say that it is impossible to get too much calcium-not toxic. Few say hypercalcemia is possible.
**Enemies-**Large quantities of fat, oxalic acid, phytic acid.
**Natural Sources-**Cheeses, soybeans, sardines, salmon, peanuts, walnuts, sunflower seeds, dried beans, green vegetables, tubers-potatoes etc., tofu, milk, milk products.
**Herb Sources-**Alfalfa, Aloe, Black Walnut, Capsicum, Cascara, Camomile, Comfrey, Dandelion, Fennel, Garlic, Ginger, Ginseng, Goldenseal, Kelp, Marshmallow, Papaya, Parsley, Poke Root, Red Clover, Red Raspberry, Rose Hips, Rosemary, Sage, Slippery Elm, White Oak Bark.

# CHROMIUM

Very small amounts of organic Chromium are found in the blood. That small amount is extremely important in aiding insulin in glucose metabolism. Chromium is the active factor in the substance GTF-glucose tolerance factor. It makes insulin more effective. In fact without Chromium insulin can't do its job. It can help prevent diabetes or hypoglycemia or help those with diabetes and hypoglycemia get by with less insulin.

As one gets older less Chromium is retained in the body. Also, a fetus may rob the Chromium stores of a pregnant women. While the body only needs trace amounts, it does need those amounts. The elderly and pregnant women, as well as those with blood sugar diseases, should obtain extra Chromium.

## Positive Effects

Aids glucose metabolism

Makes insulin more effective

Improves glucose tolerance

Restores normal insulin
levels

Transports glucose to the
cells

Deterrent for diabetes and
hypoglycemia

Prevents adult onset diabetes

Helps carbohydrate metabolism

Prevents and lowers high
blood pressure

Inhibits cholesterol formation
in liver

Reduces high blood levels
of cholesterol and triglycerides, particularly LDL
(lower density lipids)

Growth aid

Helps protein where it is
needed

**Deficiency Disease-**Suspected cause of diabetes and arteriosclerosis
**Signs of Deficiency-**Rare in most countries but it does occur in the United States. Perhaps our over refinement of food which strip essential minerals away may account for part of this.

Insulin function problems

Glucose intolerance

Arteriosclerosis

Heart cholesterol problems

Adult onset of diabetes

Diabetes and hypoglycemia

Recommended 25 mcg. /day
for healthy people with
good diets to 250 mcg.
/day if over 65 or have diabetes.

**Toxicity-**Trivalent Chromium, the kind found in food, is non-toxic and beneficial to man. Hexavalent Chromium, a pollutant found in heavy polluted areas, is toxic. Vitamin C converts it to trivalent chromium.

**Enemies-**Sugar, refined carbohydrates, refined foods, junk foods.

**Natural Sources-**Brewers yeast, whole grains, liver, mushrooms, corn and corn oil, meat, shellfish, chicken, clams, potatoes with skin, fresh vegetables, cheese, chicken legs.

**Herb Sources-**Kelp, Licorice.

# COBALT

Called the mineral that thinks it's a vitamin; thus the name cobalamin—cobalt + vitamin. It is an integral part of Vitamin $B_{12}$. Cobalamin is important for function and maintenance of body cells. It is essential for adequate red blood cell formation. Vitamin $B_6$, iron and calcium also help Cobalamin with its functions.

Most food sources that contain cobalamin are animal protein. For this reason strict vegetarians may need supplements. The body requires at least 3 micrograms a day. Suggested supplements range from 5 mcg to 25 mcg. a day depending on your diet, age and deficiency problems. 5 mcg. suggested for healthy people and up to 25 for those with suspected deficiencies. Sometimes it takes a long time to show deficiencies because the liver stores any extra cobalamin.

**Positive Effects**

Body cell maintenance and function

Healthy red blood cell production

Prevents anemia

Alert mind

Energy

Necessary for folic acid metabolism

Keeps myelin sheath from wearing thin

Metabolism of protein and essential fats

Helps carbohydrate digestion

Helps sensory motor system

Keeps glutathione active

Normal growth rate

**Deficiency Disease-**Pernicious Anemia

**Signs of Deficiency**

Poor growth rate

Fatigue

Paleness

Diarrhea

Nerves deprived of energy

Finger and toe numbness

Heart palpitations

Unsteady gait

Mind loses sharpness

Pernicious Anemia

Paralysis; if shortage goes on long enough, even death

**Toxicity-**no known toxicity.

**Enemies-**acids, alkalies, water, sunlight, alcohol, estrogen, sleeping pills.

**Natural Sources-**raw liver, liver, organ meats, beef, tuna, haddock, egg, swiss cheese, milk, cottage cheese, chicken white meat, cheddar cheese, yogurt.

Note: A deficiency is most often a result of poor absorption rather than a poor diet.

**Herb Sources-**Dandelion, Horsetail, Juniper, Kelp, Lobelia, Parsley, Red Clover, White Oak Bark.

# COPPER

A trace mineral which means only small amounts are found and needed in the body. It is thought that about 2 milligrams are needed by adults per day. Copper is important to iron metabolism. It is necessary to convert iron into hemoglobin. Copper can reach the bloodstream 15 minutes after ingesting it.

Unprocessed foods are rich in copper, unless your diet is mainly refined foods you should have no problems with copper deficiencies. Too much copper can lower the zinc levels in your body. Therefore, the best way to get sufficient copper is to eat foods containing it and let nature do the balancing. Copper assimilation is also better when Vitamin C is taken in smaller doses throughout the day rather than a large single dose.

**Positive Effects-**

Helps convert iron to hemoglobin

Important to manufacture
  of red blood cells

Coronary arteries strong

Increases energy

Helps prevent gray hair

Skin and hair pigmentation

Oxidation of Vitamin C

Bone growth and health

Protein metabolism

Taste perception

Helps nerve function-calms

Helps thinking

**Deficiency Disease-**Anemia, edema
**Signs of Deficiency-**very rare, doesn't occur alone

Anemia

Bone disorders

Pigmentation defects in
  animals

**Toxicity-**Rare, if there is too much the body usually gets rid of the excess. More than 15 mg. a day can cause unpleasant side effects: nausea, vomiting, diarrhea, intestinal cramping. Excess copper lowers zinc levels, produces insomnia, hair loss, depression and irregular menses. **It is best to get copper from food.**
**Enemies-**Too much zinc. (Copper is not easily destroyed.)
**Natural Sources-**Whole grains, almonds, leafy green vegetables, dried beans and peas, liver, eggs, prunes, oranges, beets, shrimp, most seafood.
**Herb Sources-**Burdock, Chickweed, Comfrey, Dandelion,

Echinacea, Eyebright, Garlic, Goldenseal, Horsetail, Juniper, Kelp, Lobelia, Peppermint, Red Clover, Sarsaparilla, Slippery Elm, Valerian, Yarrow.

# FLUORINE

An essential mineral. Needed in small amounts by the body though the amount needed has not been specified. It is found in bones and teeth as fluorides and helps to make them stronger.

A synthetic compound, Sodium Fluoride, is sometimes put into water of fluoridated drinking water. A natural substance, Calcium Fluoride, occurs in food. There is much controversy over Fluoride in the water, personally we are against it. We feel some are choosing their teeth over their liver.

**Positive Effects**

Reduces tooth decay                     Strengthens bones

**Deficiency Disease-**tooth decay

**Toxicity-**Doses of 20 to 80 mg. a day. Can cause problems with vitamins metabolism, discolor teeth, liver and kidney damage, damage to the central nervous system and the heart.

**Enemies-**Aluminum salts of fluoride

**Natural Sources-**Seafood, sunflower seeds, oats, garlic, gelatin, potatoes, apples, spinach and kale, wheat germ, soybeans, grapefruit, brown rice, beef, beef liver, chicken, eggs, corn.

**Herb Sources-**Alfalfa, Black Walnut, Hops, Kelp.

# IODINE

Almost all of the trace mineral Iodine goes to the thyroid gland to manufacture thyroxin. Thyroxin is a hormone that affects growth and metabolism. It is mostly made up of iodine.

Pregnant women who are deficient in iodine may give birth to babies with cretinism, a form of retardation. For this reason extra iodine is suggested for pregnant and lactating women. 100 to 150 mg. are recommended for adults and teenagers but 125-175 mg. are suggested for pregnant women and 150-200 mg. nursing women. Remember this amount can come from food not just supplements.

**Positive Effects-**

Proper function of thyroid           Helps metabolism
   gland                               Gives more energy

Helps dieting
Burns excess fat
Promotes proper growth
Healthy skin, hair, nails
  and teeth

Prevents goiter
Prevents hypothyroidism
  cretinism in newborns
  when taken by pregnant women

**Deficiency Disease-**Hypothyroidism, Goiter.
**Signs of Deficiency-**

Poor metabolism
Weight gain
Obesity
Slow mental activity
Hardening of arteries
Heart palpitations

Thick skin
Lack of energy
Cold hands and feet
Nervousness
In pregnant woman can result
  in cretinism in newborns

**Toxicity-**Natural occurring iodine is not toxic but large doses of prescription iodine can cause problems with the thyroid gland. Prescription iodine should be started gradually.
**Enemies-**Iodine poor soil, Food processing.
**Natural Sources-**Kelp, fish, all seafood, sea plants, garlic, pears, mushrooms, onions, pineapple, vegetables grown iodine-rich soil, iodized table salt.
**Herb Sources-**Kelp.

# IRON

Iron is necessary to produce hemoglobin, a protein which carries oxygen to the cells of the body and carries carbon dioxide away from the cells. Sufficient hemoglobin provides energy because the cells are receiving sufficient oxygen. Iron is also in the enzymes that play a major role in muscle function. It is necessary for proper assimilation of the B vitamins.

Calcium, copper, cobalt, and vitamin C need to be present in order for iron to do its work. Taking Vitamin C or foods containing Vitamin C with meals greatly increases the iron absorption of the food being eaten. Calcium also helps assimilation of iron. Making sure you obtain enough iron from food or a supplement is important, especially for women. **Iron and calcium are said to be the 2 major deficiencies in the diet of American women.**

Ten mg. are suggested for men and 15-18 mg. for women. More iron is required when blood loss occurs either through menstruation or through other bleeding. The elderly need additional iron because they often absorb it poorly. Pregnant women require extra iron to help maintain their iron stores and to support the growing fetus. Those who have growth spurts such as children and teenagers may also require extra iron.

**Positive Effects-**

Hemoglobin production

Prevent fatigue

Aids growth

Disease and stress resistance

Muscle functions

Good skin tone

Prevent and relieve iron-deficiency anemia

**Deficiency Disease-**Iron deficiency anemia

**Signs of Deficiency**

Anemia

Unusual fatigue

Bodily weakness

General debility

Poor endurance

Breathing troubles

Dizziness

Irritability

Hazy thinking

Flatulence

Sickly looking skin

Brittle nails

Short attention span

Depression

Overall Itching

Headaches

Sore tongue

Heartburn

Nausea after meals

Loss of appetite

Constipation or diarrhea

Hair loss

Heart palpitations

**Toxicity-**Rare, excessive doses may be harmful to children. *Hydrolized-protein chelate* supplements are organic iron and are easy to assimilate. *Ferrous* sulfate is inorganic iron. It can destroy vitamin E but can be assimilated by the body to a small degree. *Ferric* iron, a form used in many iron supplements, is like rust; it is not assimilated by the body. Both Ferric and Ferrous iron, the types that are usually put in iron enriched foods, can be deposited in the liver and can cause constipation.

**Enemies-**Phosphate food additives. E.D.T.A.-a food preservative, Tannic acid in tea, and coffee.

**Natural Sources-**Liver, blackstrap molasses, brewers yeast, sunflower seeds, dried peas and beans, eggs, oysters, lentils, prunes, raisins, dried peaches, whole grain cereals, oatmeal, wheat germ, grapes, apricots, dates, lean meat, nuts, green vegetables, (Broccoli, asparagus, spinach etc.)

**Herb Sources-**Alfalfa, Aloe, Burdock, Capsicum, Camomile, Chickweed, Comfrey, Dandelion, Echinacea, Eyebright, Fenugreek, Garlic, Ginger, Ginseng, Goldenseal, Hawthorne, Hops, Horsetail,

Kelp, Lobelia, Marshmallow, Mullein, Papaya, Parsley, Peppermint, Poke Root, Red Clover, Red Raspberry, Rose Hips, Rosemary, Sarsaparilla, Skullcap, Slippery Elm, Taheebo, White Oak Bark, Yarrow, Yellow Dock.

# MAGNESIUM

Magnesium is called the anti-stress mineral. It has calming effect when taken. It is necessary for metabolism of Calcium, Vitamin C, Phosphorus, Sodium and Potassium. Vitamin B6 helps utlization of magnesium. It is used by the body to spark energy. (See also phosphorus)

300-400 mg. are suggested daily for adults. More is needed for pregnant or nursing women.

**Positive Effects**

Helps nerve functions
Fights depression
Helps muscle functions
Lowers blood pressure
Cardiovascular system
Prevents heart attacks
Necessary for strong teeth, bones and soft tissues
Sparks energy release in body

Helps bone growth
Prevents calcium deposits
Prevents kidney and gallstones
Helps mineral metabolism
Helps acid/alkaline balance
Aids carbohydrate metabolism
Relief from indigestion
Helps turn blood sugar to energy

**Deficiency Disease-**Nervousness, extreme

**Signs of Deficiency**

Mental Confusion and disorientation
Depression
Nervousness
Easily aroused anger
Muscle tremors
Loss of appetite
Alcoholics are usually deficient

Rapid pulse
Irregular heartbeat
Blood clots in heart and brain
Coronary heart disease
Atherosclerosis
Lethargy
Nausea
Diarrhea
Malnutrition

**Toxicity-**not toxic for normal people. May give problems to those whose Calcium-phosphorus balance is off.

**Enemies-**Alcohol, diuretics, too much sugar, refined flour, too much protein, food processing.
**Natural Sources-**Soybeans, fresh green vegetables, raw wheat germ, apples, almonds, nuts, honey, peaches, brown rice, figs, lemons, grapefruit, bran, yellow corn, seeds.
**Herb Sources-**Alfalfa, Aloe, Black Walnut, Blue Cohosh, Capsicum, Catnip, Camomile, Comfrey, Dandelion, Garlic, Ginger, Gotu Kola, Hops, Kelp, Mullein, Papaya, Parsley, Peppermint, Red Clover, Rosemary, Valerian, Wood Betony.

# MANGANESE

A trace mineral. Needed for normal bone growth and structure. Catalyst for Vitamin B and C. Helps with the proper use of Vitamin E. It is important to reproduction because it aids the manufacture of sex hormones and lactation. Manganese also helps in the formation of thyroxin and in vitamin and carbohydrate metabolism.

**Positive Effects**

Skeletal growth
Muscle reflexes and co-ordination
Multiple sclerosis
Important for normal central nervous system
Improves memory
Reduces nervous irritability
May help epilepsy
Helps diabetes

Helps weak muscles and co-ordination loss
Aids digestion and food utilization
Important to production of fatty acids
Helps eliminate fatigue
Helps reproduction
Helps lactation

**Deficiency Disease-**Ataxia (loss of muscle co-ordination)
**Signs of Deficiency**

Poor muscle co-ordination
Bones bow
Poor cartilage development
Memory problems
Absentmindedness

Dizziness
Hearing problems
Ear noises
Lost ability to remove excess sugar from blood

**Toxicity-**rare-usually from industrial sources.
**Enemies-**Large phosphorus and calcium intake, heavy milk drinking and meat eating.
**Natural Sources-**Nuts, green leafy vegetables, whole grain cereals, peas, beets, egg yolks, celery, liver, banana, sweet potatoes, corn, green beans, prunes.

**Herb Sources-**Aloe, Barberry, Black Walnut, Cascara, Catnip, Camomile, Chickweed, Garlic, Goldenseal, Hops, Horsetail, Kelp, Licorice, Red Clover, Red Raspberry, Sarsaparilla, Wood Betony, Yarrow, Yellow Dock.

## MOLYBDENUM (Mol lib deh num)

A little known trace mineral. Very small amounts from 0.15 to 0.5 milligrams are needed daily by humans. Food sources are so plentiful for this mineral that supplementing is not necessary unless all the food you eat comes from nutrient-deficient soil.

Molybdenum frees iron stored in the liver so it can carry oxygen to the body cells and tissue. It works with the enzyme systems to help eliminate toxic nitrogen waste by turning it into uric acid. The uric acid can then be taken as part of urea and flushed out of the system.

**Positive Effects**

Part of iron utilization

Helps prevent anemia

Helps oxygen be carried to the body cells

Helps enzyme system of body

Promotes general well being

Aids in carbohydrate and fat metabolism

Dental enamel rich in molybdenum

May enhance effect of fluorine in tooth decay prevention

**Deficiency Disease-**none known

**Signs of Deficiency**

No deficiencies have been found in people; only in animals. However, eating large amounts of refined foods may lead to a deficiency. Whole wheat has twice the amount of molybdenum as white flour made from it.

**Toxicity-**rare. Supplements are not recommended. The best way to obtain enough molybdenum is to eat whole foods, not refined foods. Too much molydenum can lead to copper deficiency. Excessive amounts of molybdenum have been linked to gout and bone disease.

**Enemies-**Refined foods

**Natural Sources-**Leafy, dark green vegetables, whole grains, legumes (beans and peas), meat.

## PHOSPHORUS

Abundant in the body, it is present in every cell. It is thought that Phosphorus plays a role in all the chemical reactions of the body. It is one of the major parts of the teeth, in fact most of the body's Phosphorus is in the bones and teeth. Most of the *rest* of the body's Phosphorus is in the cells and body fluids in a form called ATP (adenosine triphosphate.) ATP is a substance which controls the energy release of the body. Magnesium sparks energy and Phosphorus controls it. Without Magnesium we wouldn't have any energy and without Phosphorus controlling the energy we would burn ourselves out or have to eat round the clock.

Phosphorus is essential to nerve functions especially those of nerve impulse. In fact the brain is largely made up of fats that have been chemically combined with Phosphorus.

Vitamin D and Calcium are essential for proper Phosphorus functioning. Most researchers feel taking Calcium and Phosphorus in a 1:1 ratio is best because that is the way the body uses them. However some feel that extra Calcium is necessary because Phosphorus is more easily obtained from food and because of the increased Phosphorus additives in our food and environment.

**Positive Effects**

Normal, healthy bones, teeth and gums
Aids in repair and growth
Lessens arthritis pain
Energy and vigor
Cell metabolism
Important to nerve function
Helps nerve impulse
Normal kidney function
Helps hormone production
Helps production of lecithin
Proper use of vitamins
Necessary for Niacin (Vitamin B3) assimilation
Proper sugar metabolism
Assimilation of proteins, fat and carbohydrates
Helps convert nutrients to energy
Heart regularity
Body fluids

**Deficiency Disease-**Rickets, pyorrhea, arthritis
**Signs of Deficiency**

Poor bone growth
Teeth and gum problems
Arthritis
Poor appetite control
Underweight or overweight

**Toxicity-**none known. Excesses cause Calcium to be excreted in the urine.
**Enemies-**Too much aluminum, magnesium, or iron.
**Natural Sources-**seafood, eggs, dairy products, vegetables, whole grains, nuts, seeds, meat, poultry.
**Herb Sources-**Alfalfa, Barberry, Black Cohosh, Black Walnut, Blue

Cohosh, Capsicum, Catnip, Comfrey, Dandelion, Garlic, Ginger, Goldenseal, Hawthorne, Kelp, Papaya, Parsley, Poke Root, Red Raspberry, Rosemary, Sage, Slippery Elm, White Oak Bark, Wood Betony.

# POTASSIUM

Works with Sodium to balance the body fluids, to keep the acid/ alkaline balance to those fluids, and regulate the heart beat. Potassium is necessary to move substances (nutrients, wastes etc.) through the cell walls. The body uses what has been called a Sodium-Potassium pump. Potassium works inside the cell walls and Sodium works just outside the cell walls. Potassium and Sodium are called electrolytes because they carry an electrical charge. It is this electrical charge that "goes off" and allows the two electrolytes to pump the needed substances in and out of the cell.

More potassium is needed by the body during stress, whether physical or mental stress. Also severe diarrhea, long fasts and hypoglycemia cause the body to lose potassium.

Potassium is plentiful in food, especially in whole and unrefined food, whereas Sodium is plentiful but not as plentiful as Potassium in food. The kidneys are trained to get rid of extra potassium and hoard Sodium. But man has pulled a switch on the kidneys, he is now eating less and less potassium because of refined food eating, and more and more foods containing Sodium such as potato chips, pretzels, snack type foods, etc. The kidneys are still performing their original functions of excreting extra potassium and hoarding sodium. Too much Sodium causes high blood pressure and other problems. Perhaps since we can't change our kidneys, we should change our diet back to the nutritious whole foods nature intended. Doing that would eliminate a lot more problems than just the current Sodium/Potassium imbalance.

**Positive Effects**

| | |
|---|---|
| Balances body fluids | Nutrients etc. to cell |
| Acid/alkaline balance of fluids | Helps handle stress |
| | Calms nerves |
| Regulates heart beat | Helps hypoglycemia |
| Prevents high blood pressure | Helps convert glucose into glycogen |
| Helps edema | |
| Helps oxygen transport to brain | Balances Sodium |
| | Helps body grow normally |

| | |
|---|---|
| Aids in waste elimination | Maintains healthly skin |
| Cancer deterrent | |

**Deficiency Disease-**Edema, hypoglycemia
**Signs of Deficiency-**\*Alcoholics are usually deficient

| | |
|---|---|
| Irregular heart beat | Continuous thirst |
| Heart weak or degenerate | Low blood sugar |
| Hypertension | Gas-indigestion |
| Edema | Constipation |
| Nerve and muscle disorders | Overall weakness |
| Mental and Physical stress | Sick feeling |
| Nervousness | Saggy muscles |
| Insomnia | Dry skin |
| Poor reflexes | Ear noises |
| Muscle weakness-paralysis | Poor breathing |
| General tired feeling | |

**Toxicity-**No toxic effects unless a huge dose is taken, 25 grams or more.
**Enemies-**alcohol, coffee, sugar, diuretics, refined foods.
**Natural Sources-**Blackstrap molasses, bananas, tomatoes and tomato juice, apples, grapefruit, beans, carrots, celery, citrus fruits, sunflower seeds, watercress, leafy green vegetables, mint leaves, cantaloupe, potatoes, vegetables, whole grains, nuts, fruits, apricots, dates, figs, peaches, raisins, squash, meat, fish,
**Herb Sources-**Alfalfa, Aloe, Black Walnut, Blue Cohosh, Capsicum, Cascara, Camomile, Chaparral, Comfrey, Dandelion, Echinacea, Fennel, Garlic, Ginger, Goldenseal, Kelp, Mullein, Papaya, Parsley, Peppermint, Raspberry, Rosehips, Slippery Elm, Valerian, White Oak Bark, Yarrow.

# SELENIUM

Was discovered over 20 years ago but its importance to humans is just beginning to be realized. It is present in the body in small quantities. It acts as an antioxidant and works in a synergistic relationship with Vitamin E. It has been called a catalyst. Males seem to have a greater need for Selenium than females. About half the Selenium in a man's body is found in the reproductive organs. Also, Selenium is lost in semen.

Because of the recent finding about Selenium some people take large quantities. Since such small amounts are found in the body mega-doses are probably not needed in supplements. A little goes a long way. Moderation would be advised until more research about how much is needed is available. Perhaps again a good diet of foods containing Selenium would benefit most of us and a supplement of Vitamin E with moderate amounts of Selenium would be best for those who desire supplements.

**Positive Effects**

| | |
|---|---|
| Antioxidant | Works in enzyme systems |
| Cell production against harmful oxidation including internal fats. | Helps heart function |
| | Sound and healthy muscles |
| | Stimulates antibody production |
| Keeps elasticity in tissue | Protein synthesization in |
| Prevents aging | red blood cells and liver |
| Activates DNA and RNA | Links oxygen to hydrogen |
| May neutralize some carcinogins | Menopausal distress |
| May help prevent cancer | Alleviates hot flashes |
| Growth aid | Used to treat and prevent |
| Helps some metabolic functions | dandruff |

**Deficiency Disease-**Premature aging, Premature stamina loss
**Signs of Deficiency**

| | |
|---|---|
| Premature aging | Skin problems |
| Premature stamina loss | Infertility |
| Muscular weakness and aches | Heart disease and problems |
| Pain when walking or lameness | May contribute to strokes |
| Tender thighs | |

**Toxicity-**There have been a few problems with animals grazing on lands with mostly Selenium accumulator plants (plants which suck up extra-ordinary high amounts of selenium) on them. Toxic levels are considered to be about 5 parts per million for animals and 2400-3000 micrograms daily for humans. We only need 50-200 micrograms a day unless a severe deficiency is known.

**Enemies-**Food-processing techniques, high fat foods, infection or injury stress, blood loss, old age.

**Natural Sources-**Bran, onions, tomatoes, brewers yeast, kelp, eggs, milk, wheat germ, tuna fish, broccoli.

**Herb Sources-**Garlic, Kelp, Lobelia, Red Clover, Slippery Elm.

# SODIUM

Sodium and potassium were discovered together. They work in the body to regulate the heart beat, the fluid balance, the acid/alkaline balance and others. Sodium also helps Calcium and other minerals remain soluble in the blood. (See also Potassium section)

Because of the low-sodium diet emphasis, sodium has a bad reputation. Sodium is a necessary nutrient, the body uses it in every cell. **The body simply doesn't need as much as most of our diets give it.** (some people use 10 to 35 times more than they need) Sodium is good, *excess* Sodium is not.

It is extremely difficult to buy any processed food that does not have added salt in it. Only ⅛ tsp. or less of added salt is needed **if no other salt is added to the rest of the food we eat.** Sodium is in food, you do not have to add Sodium Chloride (table salt) to obtain sodium. Perhaps it is time to begin enjoying the delicious **natural** taste of food.

Too much Sodium has been linked to edema, hypertension, and depletes the body's potassium. For excess sodium problems, a diet change is more effective than chemical diuretics because they flush out electolytes along with the water. Herbal diuretics are high in these mineral electrolytes and do not cause this flushing-out problem.

**Positive Effects**

| | |
|---|---|
| Normal growth | Muscle activity |
| Prevents heat prostration or sunstroke | Acid/alkaline balance |
| | Fluid balance of body |
| Nerve and muscle function | Aids digestion |

**Deficiency Disease-**Very rare, excess more common. Impaired carbohydrate digestion, Nerve problems.

**Signs of Deficiency**

| | |
|---|---|
| Nerve pain | Low blood sugar |
| Neuralgia | Heart degeneration |
| Indigestion and gas | Muscle shrinkage or paralysis |
| Weight loss | Arthritis |

**Toxicity-**14 grams of Sodium Chloride.

**Enemies-**Vomiting, diarrhea, sweating for fevers, heat, or excercise. May need to replace electrolytes.

**Natural Sources-**Kelp, beets, carrots, shellfish, brains, kidney, meat.

**Herb Sources-**Alfalfa, Aloe, Catnip, Chaparral, Chickweed, Dandelion, Fennel, Ginger, Hawthorne, Horesetail, Kelp, Lobelia, Marshmallow, Papaya, Parsley, Rose Hips, Rosemary, Sage, Sarsaparilla, Slippery Elm, Thyme, White Oak Bark.

# SULFUR

Sulfur the nutrient and Sulfur the pollutant emitted into the air are not the same. The nutrient, organic sulfur, is neccessary for all basic body metabolisms. It works with the B Complex vitamins and is contained in Vitamin B1, (Thiamine), Biotin and Vitamin B5 (Pantothenic Acid.) Hemoglobin contains sulfur. Sulfur is found in all body proteins; in fact, sulfur is considered a key ingredient in protein, aiding it in all its functions.

**Positive Effects**

Helps in production of collagen, building of tissue, body repair and maintenance.

Helps antibody production

Helps fight bacterial infections

Aids liver in bile secretion

Liver has many enzymes containing sulfur

Aids carbohydrate metabolism

Attaches with pollutants so they can be removed

Aids carrying of oxygen in blood

Helps maintains oxygen balance necessary for proper brain functions

Contained in Insulin, adrenalin, and thyroxin.

Youthful looking, toned skin

Smooth lustrous hair

Healthy finger and toe nails

Sulfur creams used for skin problems

**Deficiency Disease-**None known.

**Signs of Deficiency-**Reduced ability to tolerate effects of chemicals. Less resistant to poisons or drug side effects. Skin problems.

**Toxicity-**None known from organic sulfur, but ill effects may occur from large amounts of inorganic sulfur.

**Enemies-**None known.

**Natural Sources-**Fish, eggs, cabbage, dried beans, nut, radishes, brussel sprouts, soybeans, peanuts, wheat germ, meat, lean beef.

**Herb Sources-**Alfalfa, Burdock, Capsicum, Catnip, Chaparral, Comfrey, Dandelion, Echinacea, Fennel, Garlic, Juniper, Kelp, Lobelia, Mullein, Parsley, Peppermint, Sarsaparilla, Thyme, White Oak Bark.

# VANADIUM

Trace mineral. Very small amounts of this mineral go far in the body. Only about 100 to 300 micrograms (0.1 to 0.3 milligrams) are needed a day. Most Vanadium is used by the body, very little is stored. The small amount that is kept is put in the storehouse-the liver.

Vanadium has a possible role in warding off fatty plaquing or arteries.

**Positive Effects**

| | |
|---|---|
| Less arteriole plaquing | Resistance to tooth decay |
| Lowers cholesterol and tri- | Iron metabolism |
| glycerides | Red blood cell growth |
| Aids in preventing heart | Helps bone, cartilage and |
| attacks | teeth. |

**Deficiency Disease-**None known.
**Signs of Deficiency**

| | |
|---|---|
| Possible higher blood lipids | Less red blood cells |
| (cholesterol and triglycerides) | |

**Toxicity-**Yes, if in synthetic form.
**Enemies-**Not known.
**Natural Sources-**Fish, whole grains, liver, meat.
**Herb Sources-**Kelp.

# ZINC

"Zinc helps you think" or "Think Zinc"are very familiar phrases to those acquainted with this very important mineral. There are small quantities, approximately ½ teaspoon or 2½ grams, of Zinc found throughout the body. Most of this Zinc is in the muscles and bones, with the rest in the male sex organs, in the blood, skin, liver, kidneys, and pancreas. Zinc is an ingredient of insulin. Zinc is essential for all bodily processes and acts as a energy catalyst.

Copper is used like an alloy by Zinc. Taking extra zinc may require extra copper or it will be used up by Zinc. The best way to add extra copper is by eating copper rich foods. (See Copper) However, since Zinc is probably deficient in most of our diets, adding zinc supplements may be good. At least 15 mg. of zinc is needed daily by the body, 20 mg. for pregnant women and 25 mg. for nursing women.

Zinc is a mineral that is important to both men and women. Men have lots of Zinc in their prostate; in fact prostate problems can be prevented by making sure you have sufficient zinc. Women share their zinc stores with their unborn babies so it is possible for them to become depleted. Also there are some theories that Down's Syndrome may be caused in part by the mother not having enough zinc.

Those who have extra zinc needs are: the elderly, hospital patients, (especially surgery patients or those with bleeding), pregnant women, growing children, teenagers (stretch marks occur when zinc and B6 are deficient in the body), and those who lose zinc through excessive sweating.

## Positive Effects

Speeds up wound healing

Rids white spots on nails

Helps eliminate smell and
taste loss

Used with B6 prevents stretch
marks

Prevents baldness

Helps reproductive organs

Prevents infertility problems

Prevents prostate problems

Necessary for brain function

Helps decrease cholestrol
deposits

Insulin formation

Helps prevents diabetes

Helps some gum diseases

Helps crippling arthritis

Used for poison ivy

Reduces inflammation

Clears inflammatory acne

Helps prevent acrodermatitis
and Crohn's disease

Keen night vision

Reduces body odor

Schizophrenia treatment

DNA synthesis

Promotes mental alertness

Normal growth

Governs muscle contraction

Protein synthesis

Digestion

Maintains enzyme systems
and cells

Acid /alkaline balance

Blood stability

Infection resistance

**Deficiency Disease-**Possible non-cancerous enlargement of the prostate gland, arteriosclerosis.

## Signs of Deficiency

White spots on nails

Stretch marks

Growth problems

Retarded growth

Sex organs not fully developed

Prostate problems

Anemia

Liver and spleen problems

Weight loss

Listlessness

Skin sores

Rough scaly skin

Inflammatory acne

Vitamin A assimilation problems

Slow wound healing

Poor night vision

Smell loss                          Dull taste or loss
Loss of appetite

**Toxicity-**None known. Can deplete copper stores, make sure copper is sufficient in diet.
**Enemies-**Food processing, nutrient poor soil, old age, oral contraceptives, alcohol.
**Natural Sources-**Brewers yeast, wheat germ and bran, sunflower seeds, eggs, green leafy vegetables, oysters, beans, liver, spinach, peas.
**Herb Sources-**Aloe, Burdock, Camomile, Chickweed, Comfrey, Dandelion, Eyebright, Garlic, Goldenseal, Hawthorne, Hops, Kelp, Licorice, Marshmallow, Rosemary, Sarsaparilla, Slippery Elm.

# WATER

The most important nutrient for the body is water. Most of the body's weight is in water (½ to ¾%.) Water is the basic solvent of all products of digestion, it regulates body temperature, and is essential for waste removal. It helps keep all body functions working, gives energy, prevents constipation, and can be used as a diet aid by depressing the appetite if taken 20 to 30 minutes before a meal.

Dehydration is the result of extreme lack of water. **The body needs 6-10 glasses of water a day.** No other liquid can take the place of water, although juices and other liquids can help the water requirements. The body needs extra water during a fever or sickness.

# TRACE MINERALS

**Herb Sources**
Alfalfa, Black Cohosh, Black Walnut, Burdock, Cascara Sagrada, Chaparral, Dandelion, Eyebright, Hawthorne, Horsetail, Juniper Berries, Kelp, Lobelia, Parsley, Peppermint, Red Clover, Rose Hips, Sage, Sarsaparilla, Thyme, Valerian Root, White Oak Bark, Yellow Dock.

# CHAPTER 4

# *This and That*

## THIS AND THAT

**Acidolphilus**
Lactobacilli Acidophilus, a live, friendly bacteria, beneficial to man.

-quickly restores friendly bacteria in case of diarrhea, **or after an antibiotic.** Helps keep this part of the immune system strong.

-supplies a natural hydrochloric acid which aids digestion.

-reduces putrefaction caused by harmful bacteria in the large intestine.

-offsets constipation.

-essential to healthy colon. An intake of 1-3 Tb. or 2 capsules 3 times a day is beneficial in maintaining a healthy colon. Regular use helps to keep the intestines clean. Benefits all ages.

**Barley Green-**
Very nutritious, similar to Wheat Grass (See Wheat Grass), but made from Barley. Considered excellent for everything. Has been specifically used in ailments like diabetes and hypoglycemia where quick energy is needed.

**Carob-**
Highly nutritious, can be used in dessert type foods or candies. A healthy chocolate substitute. However, if you're a "chocoholic" it won't taste the same; it has its own delicious taste.

**Cell Salts-**
The cell salt theory originated with Dr. Schuessler, a medical doctor from Germany. He found there were 12 basic minerals in

each human cell. When there was a deficiency of one or more of these minerals, an imbalance was created, which inhibited the cell's assimilation of needed organic nutrition. The result was unhealthy cells and therefore an unhealthly body. Even if food was eaten that was high in mineral content the cell wouldn't assimilate it because of the imbalance within the cell.

Dr. Schuessler took natural minerals, ground them to a fine powder, then processed them to a very minute, even microscopic, energy level. In this form the mineral would bypass the digestive system and enter the weakened cell stimulating and creating a healthy cell.

These processed minerals were named cell salts. There are 12 basic salts. Dr. Schuessler found that certain cell salts treated certain symptoms, so the 12 cell salts became remedies for many ailments. Today there are herbal, vitamin, mineral, enzyme, and cell salt combinations all in one capsule. These, when combined have a synergistic effect and become a potent remedy for ailments.

**Chinese Herbal and Flower Oils-**

The Chinese are some of the greatest herbalists. They have been using herbs and handing down their remedies from generation to generation. Some of these exclusive oil formulas are now available in the U.S. The Chinese believe when one uses the oils either externally or internally they generate an energy that helps the body in healing and relieving pain. One of the main uses for oils has been for headaches, even migraines. They have also been used for: Allergies, colds, coughs, cuts, bleeding, long distance driving, motion sickness, muscle pain, and others.

**Cider Vinegar-**

The best kind of cider vinegar is the kind aged in wood, not chemically aged. It is good to have on hand as it is used in many internal and external remedies.

—a good food to add to your diet. It contains minute quantities of minerals and a mild acidity that balances and aids our digestion. The acetic acid and potassium content help to activate the good bacteria in digesting food and deter harmful bacteria in the intestines. Consequently, as we better assimilate the food we eat, we will be healthier. Has been used for arthritis, asthma, calcium assimilation, constipation, coughs (inhale in steamer), diarrhea, gout, hay fever, heartburn, laryngitis, mouthwash, rheumatism, shingles (externally and internally), sore throats.

**Enzymes-**

Enzymes are various organic substances that are produced in

plant and animal cells which cause or speed changes in other substances by catalytic action.

-help to stimulate energy and slow down the aging process. As we age the body seems less able to produce digestive enzymes. For this reason people 35 and over may need to take an enzyme supplement. Eat lots of fresh, raw foods, since heat is the enemy of enzymes and raw foods contain the highest amount of enzymes.

Dr. Earp-Thomas says "that a lack of enzymes in digestive system" promotes the growth of toxins in the colon which usually ends up in growths, tumors, ulcers, and malignant cancers.

**L-Lysine-**

An enzyme that has been found to help cold sore virus, Herpes I and II. At first sign or start of cold sore or canker one 500 mg. tablet of Lysine has been effective in preventing them from occurring. (Aloe vera also contains this enzyme.) Some people who have had troubles with cold sores and cankers all their life have started taking one lysine tablet each day and have had no more problems with them.

Excess Arginine, an amino acid, which is in large concentration in chocolate and nuts, is thought to be a contributing cause of cankers and cold sores. Lysine and Arginine balance each other. When cankers or cold sores exist Arginine is in excess and extra Lysine is needed to bring the body back in balance.

**Mineral Water-**

Organic water, from mineral wells or springs with humus beds, that contains a high concentration of minerals, naturally chelated with acids. It is one of those supplies to have on hand at all times. (This is *not* a carbonated or sparkling spring water.)

-acts as an antiseptic, antibacterial.

-relieves soreness and pain.

-is healing to wounds, ulcers, cankers.

-deters tumors, cysts, etc.

-in many remedies and used to mix herbal poultices.

-aids in glaucoma, physical imbalance, weight loss.

**Muscle Response Testing-**

Formulated by a Chiropractic Physician, Dr. George Goodheart.

-also called Applied Kinesiology or Nutritional Muscle Testing. Considered both an art and a science.

-uses acupuncture points as pressure places or indicator spots. These points are tied into different organs and parts of the body. By pushing these points and then using an indicator muscle (usually the upper arm, deltoid muscle, however sometimes a leg muscle is used) it is possible to detect and identify possible body imbalances and nutritional needs.

-has become very popular and accepted to help determine problems in the body. There are classes taught for the lay person. It is easy to use in your own home.

**Spirulina-**

Micro-algae, which is highly nutritious and an excellent source of protein, chlorophyll, vitamins and minerals and amino acids. It has 26 times the calcium of milk, contains phosphorus, B12, RNA and DNA, and easily digested. It is a safe food with no side effects. It would be good for survival purposes as it is easy to store. Has sometimes been called "Manna of the future." It has been tested in Japan and Europe and found to benefit people who suffer from many ailments including: anemia, cataracts, diabetes, gastrointestinal disorders, glaucoma, hepatitis, physical imbalances, aids weight loss.

**Wheat Grass or Wheat Grass Juice-**

Wheat is grown to about 7 inches, then cut close to root or pulled out of sod (root can also be used). It can be chewed to extract the juice or the juice extracted with a meat grinder or wheat juicer. It is considered a complete food, is high in chlorophyll (See Chlorophyll), contains every known vitamin, high in enzymes, and over 100 elements have been identified in it. It is used in the body as a cleanser, rebuilder and neutralizer of toxins. It is a tonic, acts as a detergent in the body, and has been used for *all* ailments, some of which are listed: Anemia, Blood pressure, Cancer, Constipation, Douches, Eczema, Enemas, Hair color, Headaches, Heart, Intestines, Scars in lungs, Muscle fatigue, Poultices, Psoriasis, Colon putrification, Skin problems, Stomach aches, Toothache, Sore throat.

# CHAPTER 5

# Cleansing, Diets, and Fasts

## HOW TO CLEANSE

Imagine the filth in a house that hadn't been cleaned for 10, 20, or 50 years. Yet, we expect our bodies to keep right on functioning without ever cleaning its house. Fortunately, our body does some housecleaning by itself.

The body becomes an eliminating organ when it needs to get rid of toxic matter. The flu with its vomiting, diarrhea, and fever are good examples of the tools the body uses to expel and destroy disease. During a cold, mucus starts to flow, with sneezing, coughing, and sometimes a fever. Again the body is using its tools to rid itself of the disease.

Many people who don't understand the body's natural way to cleanse itself feel that these eliminating symptoms are all bad and should be stopped. They run for antibiotics, antihistamines, or drugs that stop diarrhea. Antibiotics not only kill the bad bacteria but also the friendly bacteria. Antihistamines stop the mucus from being eliminated from the head and keep it there so the body must try harder the next time to get rid of it. The anti-diarrhea drugs stop more than the colon eliminating; they stop the whole body eliminating process.

Health specialists say that there is only one disease—**constipation.** Not just constipation or clogging of the colon, but clogging of all internal organs. The body uses the colon as one of its chief waste disposal plants. When the colon is clean and working properly the rest of the body including organs are free to clean house" and

**151**

"dump" into the colon. If the colon is clogged the glands and organs become bogged down with toxins and unwanted mucus, some of them cease or nearly cease functioning. In many cases the result is removal of the gland or organ by surgery. There is a **better way.** A program of herbs, vitamins, minerals, diet, exercise, cleansing fasts, and enemas or colonics will help the body eliminate the toxic matter that becomes lodged in the organs and glands. These organs and glands cleanse and are able to start functioning again. A clean gland or organ is healthy.

# ELIMINATING CRISES

There are two eliminating crises the body naturally goes through to heal itself. If we understand what is going on we can **help** the body eliminate the poisons and wastes. The first is called a **Healing Crisis** and the second is called a **Disease Crisis.**

### Healing Crisis

1. Happens only when the body is strong enough to go through a cleanse, either because the body is ready to cleanse or because the body has been put on a cleansing diet.
2. Although your body may have many physical symptoms, you usually feel positive or happy.
3. Usually lasts 2 or 3 days.

### What to expect in a healing crisis

— You will probably feel like you have the flu because the body will start to eliminate toxins and poisons. (Enemas are important)
— The symptoms you have will also depend on your own particular weaknesses. For example, if you have sinus problems, you may have a lot of mucus from your head to eliminate. Or if you have bronchial problems, you may need to expel mucus from your lungs. Since everyone is different a healing crisis will affect everyone a little differently.
— By taking proper care of body; the body may cleanse itself a little at a time, bit by bit, and no crisis is necessary. Homemade soups, steamed vegetables, fresh vegetables juices, fruit juices, the herbs related to the particular area and enemas are some of the best ways to help your body through a healing crisis.
**Note:** Vegetables and vegetable juices can be used to slow down a cleanse, if the body is cleansing too fast.

**Disease Crisis**

1. Happens when the body has chronic problems after many years of not being allowed to eliminate toxins and wastes.
2. Happens when the body is full of mucus, and germs are multiplying.
3. Happens out of survival for the body to save itself.
4. Happens when the body is not strong.
5. Lasts from 2 to many weeks.
6. Besides having physical symptoms, the mental state of the body is also negative. A feeling of being very depressed is common.

**What to expect in a Disease Crisis**

1. Fever and all the symptoms of the disease. (The eliminating tools of the body.)
2. Feelings of depression.

Enemas or colonics are very important in a disease crisis to send toxins and poisons out of the body rapidly so more toxins and waste can come into the eliminating organs and be expelled.

During this time, it is very important to feed the body the type of food that will best nourish it and help it get well. (This is not a time for cheating or eating junk food.) Fresh fruits and fruit juices tend to speed up a cleanse—so when one is already very ill it is better to use mostly vegetable juices.

(See also Foods for Acute Illness, Ailments Chapter)

## THE MILD FOOD DIET

The Mild Food Diet is used in chronic illnesses when the body needs maximum nutrition with easy-to-digest foods; to help bring on or initiate a healing cleanse, or to help slow down a disease crisis, so you won't become too ill or cleanse too fast.

The diet consists of:
1. All fruits: raw or frozen, including papaya, mangos, etc.
2. Vegetables: raw as much as possible, when cooked, only lightly steamed. Bake all starch vegetables. Suggestion for tossed salads: leaf lettuce (no head lettuce), raw yams (sliced or grated), romaine lettuce, spinach, chard, raw corn, green peppers, cabbage (purple and green), grated carrots, raw beets grated, raw asparagus, zuccini, sprouted lentils, other sprouts (especially alfalfa sprouts), tomatoes, cucumbers, celery, avocado, raw or frozen peas. Also vegetable soups.

3. Fruit Juices: fresh, frozen or canned.
4. Vegetable Juices: all raw (carrot, spinach, etc.)
5. Cold pressed oils and apple cider vinegar, aged in wood, with herb seasonings for dressing for salads.

## The "no no's" of the Mild Food Diet are:

| | | |
|---|---|---|
| No refined foods | Butter | Meat |
| Grain | Eggs | Peanuts |
| Sugar | Dried legumes | Chips |

Think of what you can eat and not what you can't. You'll probably be hungry at first. Eat all the food you want as long as it is on the diet. Everything is low calorie and high nutrition.

After about 4-12 weeks your body should start a healing crisis. You will feel like you have the flu or a cold for 2 to 3 days. Keep eating the steamed vegetables and soups like you have been and take enemas (see enema section) for a couple of days to help the body cleanse. Little by little the body will build, heal and cleanse, and build, heal and cleanse until it climbs up the healing ladder to optimum health. The scale of getting better looks like this.

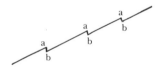

a. feel better than usual
b. healing crisis the next day for 2 or 3 days

This is called the reverse healing process. You are retracing the path you went down as you became ill in the first place. Some days on the crisis times you may feel sick enough to think you are getting worse, not better. The body is eliminating toxins and poisons, but you should start to notice that the lows are not low as they used to be and the highs are getting higher. Most experienced health people will tell you there is a time of feeling worse before getting better.

Everyone always asks, "How long will this take?" The answer is: "As long as it takes **your** body to start feeling better." If it is a chronic disease that has been going on for years it will take more time than an acute problem. This of course depends on how strong your body is, how fast your body cleanses, and how diligent you are.

If you are coming off a cleanse add the foods from the Real Food Diet slowly so your body has time to adjust to the change.

# DIET TIPS

Changing your diet is sometimes overwhelming, therefore, these tips may make it easier. The two most important things to change in your diet, and maybe the two easiest are white sugar and white flour. Use whole wheat flour instead of white flour. Use honey or molasses instead of white sugar. You will be amazed how easy you can adapt your method of cooking without even changing what you eat. This change alone if no other one were made would be tremendous in the terms of your better health.

Another step and one that is quite easy is to read labels for harmful or unnecessary additives. Look for things like BHT, BHA, MSG-monosodium glutonate, artificial colorings and flavorings, nitrates, salt, sugar or things ending in "ose" like dext*rose*, and other artificial preservatives.

Unless you are very ill and have no choice, make gradual changes that you can live with; not overnight radical changes that you are going to throw away in disgust in two or three months. Be on the look out for ways you can improve your diet that fit you and your personality. For instance, is it easy to add more vegetables or fruits to your diet. Try some low-fat cooking methods of cooking the same food you already eat.

Try to add fresh vegetables and fruits, whole grains and cereals instead of "instant" foods. In other words go back to eating "Real Food."

# REAL FOOD DIET

## Beverages

| Foods Allowed | Foods to Avoid |
|---|---|
| 1. *All herb teas* (comfrey, peppermint, alfalfa, etc.) | 1. Alcohol |
| 2. *Fresh or frozen juices* without sugar, (apple, pear-grape, grape, pineapple, etc.) | 2. Cocoa |
| | 3. Coffee |
| | 4. Carbonated beverages |
| | 5. Canned and pasteurized juices |
| 3. *Fresh vegetable juices* (carrot, green drinks, etc.) | 6. Artificial drinks |
| 4. *Carob drinks* | 7. Sugared juices or drinks |
| 5. *Chlorophyll drink* | |

6. *Vegetable broth*

Note: Carob can be substituted for chocolate. It doesn't taste like chocolate, it has its own delicious taste. It is easy to get used to and is very nutritious. Chocolate inhibits the assimilation of calcium.

## DAIRY PRODUCTS

| Foods Allowed | Foods to Avoid |
|---|---|
| 1. Raw milk, goat milk | 1. Pasteurized Milk |
| 2. Buttermilk | 2. All processed and imitation |
| 3. Nonfat cheese and white | butter. |
| cheese | 3. Ice cream and toppings |
| 4. Homemade ice cream | 4. All orange and colored, |
| with honey. | pasteurized cheeses. |
| 5. Lowfat cottage cheese | |
| 6. Lowfat yogurt with | |
| no sugar. Can put fresh | |
| fruit over it or in it. | |

Note: Goat milk is naturally homogenized and is easily assimilated. Raw cow's milk contains enzymes to help the milk be digested, these enzymes are destroyed by pasteurization. Raw milk also is less mucus forming.

## PROTEIN

| Foods Allowed | Foods to Avoid |
|---|---|
| Eggs | Eggs |
| Poached, boiled, scrambled, or in omlets. Do not fry. | Fried eggs |
| Fish | Fish |
| Fresh white-flesh, salmon, rainbow trout, or fish with fins. Broiled or baked. | Breaded or fried fish, especially deep fried fish, and shell fish. |
| Meats | Meats |
| Skinned chicken and turkey. Eat sparingly, meats are harder to digest and use more body energy to be digested. | Pork, beef, all prepared meats, (sausage, cold cuts, weiners, hams etc.) Note: Beef raises the body temperature. Pork takes at least 9 hours to be digested. Prepared meats have chemicals |

| Foods Allowed | Foods to Avoid |
|---|---|
| | that are harmful to the body. |
| Nuts and Seeds | Nuts |
| All raw and fresh, especially almonds, sunflower seeds, sweet apricot pits, pumpkin seeds, sesame seeds, etc. | Roasted and salted. Peanuts are high in acid. |

# CARBOHYDRATES

| Foods Allowed | Foods to Avoid |
|---|---|
| Grains | Grains |
| Whole grain cereals, breads, muffins, pie crusts, etc. (oats, wheat, bran, buckwheat, millet, brown rice, rye, barley, etc.) Seeds (sesame, pumpkin, sunflower, flaxseed, etc). Noodles and macaroni made from whole wheat, spinach, etc. | White flour products, hulled grains and seeds, white rice, prepared mixes and foods, cold cereals, cooked seeds. All refined or processed grains. Noodles and macaroni from white flour products. |
| Vegetables | Vegetables |
| All vegetables. Be daring, try some new ones. Some like raw yams are surprisingly delicious. Raw vegetables are the best. Use fresh or frozen vegetable and when you cook them steam or bake them. | All commercial canned vegetables, fried and deep fried vegetables, potato and corn chips, etc. |
| Fruit | Fruit |
| All fruit. Fresh, frozen, stewed, dried, unsulfured. Eat sparingly of citrus fruits, except lemons. | Candied or sugared fruits. |

# FATS

| Foods Allowed<br>Oils | Foods to Avoid<br>Oils |
|---|---|
| Cold processed oils, margarine, (if safflower or corn oil) | Saturated oils and fats, and high fat foods. |

# OTHER

| Foods Allowed | Foods to Avoid |
|---|---|
| Soups | Soups |
| All homemade. Vegetable, sprouted lentils, sprouted beans, barley, brown rice, millet, chicken broth. | Canned and creamed soups, commercial bouillon, fat stocks. |
| Sprouts | Sprouts |
| All kinds, including-alfalfa, wheat, lentil, mung, radish, cabbage, bean, etc. | none |

Note: Sprouts are the highest form of nutrition. It has been found that the time in a plant's life when it starts to sprout is the time when it contains as much as 10 times the concentration of vitamins and minerals.

| Sweets | Sweets |
|---|---|
| Raw honey, unsulfured molasses, carob, pure maple syrup, pineapple juice, apple juice or apple juice concentrate, sorghum, barley sweetener, fructose, carrots. | Refined sugars (white or brown), chocolate, candy, syrups, dextrose, sucrose, etc. |
| Seasonings | Seasonings |
| Herbs, garlic, onion, chives, parsley, majoram, capsicum, kelp, mineral or sea salt, vegetable seasoning or broth. | Black pepper, processed salt, MSG-monosodium glutamate, food enhancers or colors, etc. |

# JUICE FASTS

After being on the mild food diet or Real Food Diet, you may want to try a juice fast. We like to do one about twice a year, but it can be done every three months if necessary.

It is one of the safest and quickest ways of helping the body eliminate all kinds of toxic matter. During the juice fast, the process of elimination of dead and dying cells is speeded up and the amino acids from these old diseased cells are set free to be used in an accelerated process of building new and healthy cells. Dr. Otto Buchinger, M.D., calls juice fasting "a burning of rubbish." After the first three days on a juice fast the body burns and decomposes the most "inferior" and "impure" materials. Also at this time the eliminating organs function at a higher capacity to expel accumulated wastes and toxins. This is because the energy usually being used to digest foods is now channeled into eliminating the waste. By drinking juices, the food has already been changed so that it can be easily utilized by the body. Juices are fresh and have a concentration of vitamins and minerals.

We do not recommend long fasts, somewhere between 3 to 7 days is best. Some people start on fasts and stay on them for long periods of time or go on a fast and then off for a few days and then on again. We do not recommend this type of fasting. **Fasting should be used in moderation, to help the body cleanse, not as a replacement diet for food.** One very major reason for this is because the colon was meant to handle bulk. When the bulk is taken away for long periods of time the colon, which is only a muscle in the body, atrophies from lack of use. Many times after extremely long fasts, it is hard for the colon to begin to function properly again.

**Why Fast**

1. Chronic illness-helps to restore health.
2. General cleansing of the digestive system, lymphatic system, glandular system.
3. Toning of all cells and glands, and rejuvenating or revitalizing the body.
4. To eliminate hardened material in joints and muscles. (Arthritis, Gout etc.)
5. To lose weight.
6. For those who need to gain weight, it helps to normalize metabolism of the thin person and revitalize and clean digestive systems so they can assimilate food better.

7. To cleanse blood vessels of plaque and build good blood.

## What to Expect

1. Hunger the first 3 days. Also the first three days are usually the hardest for most people, so be patient. Drink as often as needed. Your body will probably start to feel hungry for solid food somewhere between the 5th and 7th day.

2. You should be able to keep up with your regular work and exercise.

3. You may have some dizziness or headaches as the toxins start to move into the system to be eliminated. The best thing to do if this happens is to take an enema as the wastes need to be moved out of the system.

4. You will probably feel better, have more energy and the senses become sharper during a fast than at any other time.

## How to go on a Juice Fast

— It is important to take at least one cleansing enema a day as the colon will not have the bulk needed to move the waste out. An enema morning and night is best. It is also important to exercise and get plenty of rest.

— You will need to invest in a juicer. They are well worth the investment as you will want to use fresh juices daily with your regular diet as well as for juice fasts.

— Drink as much as you want. Drink fruit juices 20 to 30 minutes apart from vegetable juices. Never mix fruit and vegetable juices except for apple or pineapple in the green drink.

You will find many kinds of juice fasts. This Variety Juice Fast is our favorite. Drink as often as desired from the following choices.

## Variety Juice Fast

1. raw apple juice
2. green drink (see recipe)
3. other fresh or frozen juices
4. carrot juice
5. herb teas
6. vegetable broths
7. chlorophyll drink (see recipe)
8. distilled or pure water
**No citrus, except lemon.**

Note: Hypoglycemics may want to dilute fruit juices with water 50/50.

## The Green Drink

1 cup raw apple or pineapple juice in blender
Add any of 4 or 5 following

| | |
|---|---|
| Parsley | Dandelion leaves |
| Celery Leaves | Spinach leaves |
| Comfrey | Marshmallow leaves |
| Beet Greens & | Spearmint-Peppermint |
| 1 small beet if desired | leaves |

Blend well—then finish filling with apple or pineapple juice. Strain for juice fast. If too sweet, add water to taste.

## Chlorophyll Drink

1 tsp. commercial concentrated chlorophyll to 1 cup water.

## Lemon Juice/Maple Syrup

Lemon juice and pure maple syrup contain many vitamins and minerals that help the body cleanse and revitalize itself. This fast is especially good to break up mineral and protein deposits in the body. It is also used for weight loss. The one on the left was originated by Stanley Burroughs.

Drink 8 to 12 glasses of the lemon/maple syrup mixture a day. A gallon can be made at a time if desired. Distilled water can be drunk in between lemon juice if desired. Peppermint tea can also be used during this fast.

2 T fresh lemon juice
2 T pure maple syrup    or
1/10 tsp. cayenne
10 oz. pure or distilled
  water.
  (Stanley Burroughs)

4 oz. lemon juice
¼ C. to ⅓ C. pure maple
  syrup  ⅓ Cup if weight
  gain is desired)
⅛ tsp. cayenne
1 qt. pure or distilled
  water.

## How to break a fast

Breaking the fast is very important. Do not overeat! Consider it part of your fast. Continue to drink juices but cut down the number of glasses as you add solid foods. The following solid foods can be added.

First Day—          Breakfast: half apple
                         Lunch: homemade vegetable soup

Second Day—                    Breakfast: half apple, or mild fruit, stewed fruit.
                               Lunch: homemade vegetable soup
                               Dinner: small vegetable salad (use leaf lettuce, not iceberg), small baked potato.
Third Day—                     Breakfast: same as second day
                               Lunch and Dinner: can start adding small portions of cottage cheese, baked potato, yogurt, whole grain bread.
Fourth Day—                    Start on Real Food Diet.

# BALANCED BODY CHEMISTRY

A balanced body chemistry is what is called a proper alkaline-acid ratio. If the body becomes over-acid, immunity to disease is weakened. It is now believed that one of the basic causes of disease is acidosis or over-acidity.

As foods are digested in the body, they leave a residue or ash which is either neutral, acid, or alkaline. Acidosis occurs when the alkaline reserve in the body is diminished.

A healthy body usually has alkaline reserves which help keep the acid balance in check. If we eat too many acid producing foods we become over-acid and are less able to resist disease. The ratio in a healthy body is 4 parts alkaline to 1 part acid. In order to keep the acid-alkaline ratio in balance, Dr. Ragnar Berg, the world's foremost authority on the subject, says that we should eat about 80 alkali producing foods and 20 acid producing foods.

Alkalis help to neutralize the acids when one does become over acid or ill. Eating more alkaline-ash foods helps the body to heal and regain its balanced chemistry.

| *Alkali Forming Foods* | *Acid Forming Foods* |
|---|---|
| Vegetables | Most grains (except millet) |
| Fruits | Buckwheat |
| Green drinks | Meats |
| Juices | Eggs |
| Broths, Soups, etc. | Nuts (except almonds) |
| Cottage cheese, Buttermilk | Lentils |

Note:   Seeds and grains become more alkaline when sprouted.

*Neutral or near Neutral*
Butter, Milk, Cream, Honey, Dried legumes.

# CHAPTER 6

# Did You Say Enema?

## DID YOU SAY ENEMA?

When the head, sinuses, and respiratory organs are full of mucus, the whole digestive system is full of mucus too. As the colon is cleaned, the rest of the body's glands and organs can start to eliminate the poisons and toxins into the colon and kidneys to be eliminated. Until the colon is cleaned out, there is no place for the other toxins to move. A congested colon becomes a breeding place for parasites (Parasites of one form or another are common) and spawning place for disease, so that is where the housecleaning of the body should start.

When people first start learning about herbs, they like them as an alternative instead of drugs. But as soon as enemas are mentioned—"Did you say enema?" However, survival is a great teacher. Reluctant feelings about enemas are overcome by a desire to live and be well. Enemas are an effective way to help overcome disease.

*Use Enemas or Colonics For:*
1. Illnesses-chronic or acute (disease or healing crisis.)
2. Fevers-tepid water and herbal enemas (see Herbal Enemas this chapter.)
3. During juice fasts.
4. Any symptom of constipation (including diarrhea.)
5. Colon diseases.
6. Colon cleanses (to clean colon of parasites, mucus, toxic material, hardened matter on colon wall.)

7. To help restore peristaltic action.
8. To help body glands and organs cleanse.
    Many ailments clear up when the colon is cleansed.

### Why cleansing colon helps.

-The body will be able to digest and utilize its food better. One of the colon's functions is to separate matter that is still nutritious from waste matter. Over the years if one has eaten processed food, enriched white flour products, greasy food, white sugar etc. the lining of the small and large intestines become coated and packed with hard old matter. Mucus and parasites become housed in pockets in the colon. The action of the colon is greatly diminished and poor elimination is the result. Then, the very best of diets cannot be utilized.

—When different places of the colon related to the other areas and organs of the body are bogged down with mucus, toxic matter and/or parasites those organs and areas are also affected. This is because the colon is related to every cell in the body and nerve endings from all parts of the body are attached to the colon.

### How to Cleanse the Colon

1. Enemas or colonics.
2. Herbal laxatives—act as a stimulant to the bile instead of an irritant to the colon lining.
3. Herbs—used as colon scrubs or brooms such as alfalfa, psyllium, comfrey/pepsin, fennel.
4. Chlorophyll drink or green drink which help soften hard matter attached to colon wall.
5. Exercise—very important since the colon is a smooth muscle and can become more efficient if it is stimulated by exercise.
6. Juice fasts accompanied by enemas.

### There are several therapies of colon cleanses:

1. *Colon Cleanse the Easy Way,* by Vena Burnett and Jennifer Weis.
2. *The Colon Health Handbook,* by Robert Gray.

It is not only important to have a clean, efficient colon for nutrition and the body's health in general, but also for the health of the colon itself. Colon diseases are becoming more prevalant in our society, some of which include Colitis, Spastic Colons, Prolapsed Colons, Redundant (elongated) colons, Diverticulitis, Constipation, Diarrhea, Hemorrhoids, and Colon cancer.

## Signs of an Unclean Colon

1. Bad breath
2. Bad body odor
3. Bad or Putrid Smell of fecal matter
4. Flatulence—Gas
5. Digestive Problems
6. Acne
7. Excess mucus in head, throat,lungs.
8. Kidney Infection
9. Prostate Problems etc.
10. Female Problems
11. Liver—Gall Bladder
12. Chronic Illness

## How to take a High Enema

We use a hospital disposable bag that is a clear plastic. They last about 6 months or so and are easily cleaned and quite inexpensive.

—For adults the knee-chest position is the easiest for insertion and also for allowing gravity to help the enema solution to flow into the entire colon area. Another position for administering enemas to elderly adults is to have them lie on their backs on a slightly elevated slant board. (4 to 6 inches) Caution: those who have high blood pressure should not use this position but can lie on their left side flat on the floor. Sometimes putting feet up on the wall will help one to retain solution.

—It is good to **gently** massage the colon during an enema. Start on the left side of the abdomen and work down in the direction of the rectal opening. As the colon is gradually emptied move over to the middle section (transverse colon) of the colon above the navel, and massage moving again in the direction of the rectal opening. Next move on the right side and work up to the transverse colon (center) again and back down the left side. Massage with enemas can help break loose hard matter easier and loosens blockages.

—Lubricate end of the tube with petroleum jelly or vitamin E. Insert the tube a few inches into the rectum past the sphincter muscle; do not force. Take only as much as is comfortable, then expel. It is important to expel when there is a need rather than try to hold more solution. Forcing yourself to hold more can sometimes balloon the colon. Allow water to flow until there is a cramp or the need to expel. As the colon becomes cleansed it will be able to hold more solution at a time, even as much as a whole bag. If the water stops flowing, slide the tube back and forth a little or start and stop the water to try to dislodge the blockage. (Massage also)

This process should be repeated until *3 bags of solution have been used.* Warm water can be used in the first two bags to help loosen hard impacted matter. Tepid to cool water can be used in the last bag to help tone the colon. Each time the solution flows in, it should go a little farther into the colon until on the last bag the entire colon should be reached.

It takes anywhere from 30 to 45 minutes for a high enema.

### For babies and children

The same process is used for children with smaller amounts: For babies ¼ bag, small children 1 bag, other children 1-2 bags depending on their size and need. Children do not take one whole bag at once, their colon is too small. Allow them to expel when they feel the need. They shouldn't have to try to take more.

Babies can be laid on a towel (see also Baby section) in the tub and very slowly allow water to enter. The baby will expel when it needs to. We use 1 pt. for babies. Remember the solution is never forced all at once but only the amount that is comfortable.

### Herbal Enemas

Distilled or purified water is most preferred for enemas. It is good to use water in the first two bags, then the herbal solution in the last bag.

| | |
|---|---|
| **Garlic-** | Especially good to fight infection anywhere in body, |
| **Why-** | pulls mucus from colon, kill parasites, for hypertension and a general cleanser of colon. |
| | Blend: 5 or 6 garlic buds to 1 Cup water. Strain. |
| **How-** | Add enough water to this to make enough solution to fill 1 enema bag. (2qts.) Or make 3 times this solution for 3 bags. If fresh garlic is not available use 8 capsules or 1 tsp garlic powder (not the kind you buy in a grocery store) to a bag. |
| | For babies we use 1 small garlic bud to 1 pint. |
| | |
| **Catnip-** | Used for fevers, contagious diseases and colic. Very |
| **Why-** | Relaxing to the entire system. Use only *tepid* water for fevers. |
| | For 2 qt. enema bag—2 heaping Tb. Catnip leaves |
| **How-** | in a container that holds a quart or more. Pour 1 Qt. boiling water over it. Let steep for 20 to 30 minutes. Strain. Add the rest of the water to the bag after tea is steeped. **If using for a fever**, let cool or add cold water to the bag to get desired tepid temperature. |

| | |
|---|---|
| **Catnip/Garlic-** | Combines positive qualities of both garlic enemas |
| **Why-** | and catnip enemas in the same enema. Garlic fights infection; pulls mucus; kills germs, bacteria, virus, and parasites; and increases peristaltic action of the colon. Catnip helps ease cramping of the colon; brings down fevers; pulls mucus; helps stop pain; and relaxes and soothes the whole system. |
| | Make a solution for a Garlic enema. (See Garlic Enema.) |
| **How-** | Make Catnip tea according to the directions given under Catnip enemas. Combine the garlic solution and the Catnip in equal parts in the enema bag. |

| | |
|---|---|
| **Cayenne-** | Stimulates kidneys, liver, spleen, and pancreas. |
| **Why-** | Also good for bleeding hemorrhoids. |
| **How-** | Add 1 tsp. or 4 capsules to a 2 qt. bag. |

| | |
|---|---|
| **Slippery Elm-** | Used for diarrhea, hemorrhoids, and colitis. Very |
| **Why-** | healing to scalded colon walls as a result of diarrhea. |
| | 1 Tb. powdered Slippery Elm in blender with 2 cups |
| **How-** | water. Add water to finish filling 2 quart bag. |

| | |
|---|---|
| **Mineral Water-** | Used for pulling toxins, mucus, parasites, general |
| **Why-** | cleansing. Tones and heals colon walls. |
| | 1/3 to 1/2 Cup to 2 quart bag of water. Note: this |
| **How-** | solution sometimes cramps a little. |

| | |
|---|---|
| **Aloe Vera-** | |
| **Why-** | Healing to colon walls, hemorrhoids, bleeding, etc. |
| **How-** | 1/3 to 1/2 Cup to 2 quart bag of water. |

# COLONICS

A colonic is an enema given by a professional colonic therapist. It is much more efficient than a regular enema as 20 to 30 gallons of water are allowed to flow freely, by gravity through the colon.

The procedure is really quite comfortable since water circulates through the colon and no pressure is built up because of retaining water before you can expel. The client lies modestly covered on a comfortable mat while the colonic therapist massages the abdominal area to loosen toxic matter. The body is covered by a large towel or sheet, so there is no embarrassment. Sometimes there is some cramping as old fecal matter, pockets of mucus and parasites break loose.

It is good to take colon cleansers during a colonic program and get daily exercise. The colon is a muscle, exercise helps tone it and helps it to become healthier. It is also important to take acidolphilus daily during a colonics program. Because of the volume of water used the friendly bacteria needs to be replaced.

The number of colonics needed depends on how toxic and impacted the colon has become. Some people only need the minimum recommended series of 3 colonics a week apart, others need 6, others take colonics for many months. The reason a series of 3 is recommended as a minimum is because the 1st colonic empties the colon and starts the body cleaning and dumping into the colon. The second colonic removes the toxins the body has pulled after the first colonic. The third does the same for the second. The reason this is not an endless cycle is because many times after these three colonic enough toxins has been removed to allow the body to efficiently deal with what is left.

For the most effective colonic, chose a therapist who stays with you during the therapy.

When a series of colonics are taken it stimulates the rest of the body to cleanse and start dumping its waste. It will sometimes bring on some cleansing reactions. These reactions may be a clue to extend the time between colonics to longer than a week until the body catches up with the colon.

It is often good to take a colonic at the beginning of an acute illness or a juice fast and then follow with some herbal enemas.

# CHAPTER 7

# *Before, During and After (Pregnancy)*

## BEFORE, DURING, AND AFTER
## (Pregnancy)

### "BEFORE"

The most important gift to give a baby is a healthy mother *before* she becomes pregnant. Women become very conscious of their health after they are pregnant, but before pregnancy they often do not take very good care of themselves. Many problems of morning sickness, iron deficiencies, fatigue, etc. could be prevented for the mother; and a healthier body and mind could be provided for the infant, if women and young girls consistently built and strengthened their bodies before marriage and pregnancy.

The healthier a woman's body is before she gets pregnant not only has a direct bearing on how she feels during the pregnancy, but also gives her baby a better start in life. In fact, in recent studies it has been found that when a woman takes a one-a-day multiple vitamin even just one month *before* pregnancy, her baby has increased neurological benefits.

The following are some suggestions of how to prepare for a pregnancy.

**How to help prepare for a pregnancy**

**Diet**—Nutrition for pregnancy begins before the pregnancy. A healthy diet is a good habit to acquire early in life. However, if you plan to try to become pregnant, it is beneficial to go on a juice fast or mild food diet to cleanse the body. The cleaner the liver and colon area, the less chance there is for nausea and hormonal imbalances. After the juice fast or mild food diet the Real Food Diet which includes many fresh fruits, vegetables, and sprouts will also help to lessen the chances of nausea or other problems. In fact many women who have problems becoming pregnant, are able to conceive after going on a juice fast or mild food diet cleanse.

**Exercise** before pregnancy is also important as it increases circulation, regulates calcium and hormonal imbalances, and in general tones the entire body, including the uterus, so delivery will be easier.

**Herbs.** A baby can inherit weaknesses from its parents. A mother can lessen this by improving any problems or weaknesses she has *before* pregnancy.

# "DURING"

(Pregnancy)

**Diet**—Real Food Diet, green drink is also important.

**Exercise**—Not a time to start a vigorous, **new** exercise program, but you can usually continue any program you are used to for most of your pregnancy. If you haven't exercised before becoming pregnant and now wish to enjoy its benefits, walking and swimming are wonderful. There are lots of books written on exercise, many of them talk about exercise during pregnancy.

### Basic Herbs for Pregnancy

1. Red Raspberry Tea—high in iron, guards against hemorrhaging, tones uterus, shorter labor. 2 capsules 3 times a day or a quart of tea a day has been used.
2. Other teas—Alfalfa, Comfrey, Mints.
3. Blood Builder Combination #1—(Kelp, Dandelion, Alfalfa)
   a. *Kelp* is high in vitamins, minerals and trace minerals. There have been tests showing it guards against fetus abnormalities.
   b. *Dandelion* has been used to prevent or correct anemia and is an excellent liver cleanser as well as being high in Vitamin and Mineral content.
   c. *Alfalfa* contains 8 essential amino acids of good digestion and helps nausea during pregnancy. Also high in Vitamin, Mineral content.
4. Calcium Combinations—help with extra calcium demands.
5. Chlorophyll or Green drink—Helps to purify and clean blood, guards against anemia, very nutritious. (See Chlorophyll)

*Case History:*

O. was in her second month of pregnancy when she began hemorrhaging. She spent two weeks in the hospital flat on her back. The bleeding slowed down a little. They told her to go home and stay down. She took 16 capsules of Red Raspberry a day; the bleeding stopped within two days.

## Daily Vitamin/Mineral and Herbal Supplements—

1. Natural multiple vitamin and mineral supplement.
2. B Complex
3. Vitamin C
4. Vitamin E

Note: Extra B, C, and E are needed at the beginning and end of pregnancy to strengthen the placenta, amniotic bag and skin tissue.

5. Calcium

Note: Extra calcium is needed during pregnancy to supply the extra demands of the fetus in building strong bones and teeth. In the mother it helps calms nerves, stops leg cramps (charley horses), and alleviates insomnia. The need for extra calcium increases even more at end of pregnancy.

## Remedies for common problems of pregnancy

## Anemia—

Blood Builder Combinations #1 & #2

| | | |
|---|---|---|
| Alfalfa | Dandelion | Yellow Dock |
| Cayenne | Kelp | |
| Chlorophyll | Red Beet | |

Iron is important for normal hemoglobin formation and carries oxygen from lungs to *every* cell in body. Taking herbs high in iron and also dandelion which normalizes the blood salts has been used to prevent or correct anemia very quickly. (See Dandelion and Yellow Dock) Most synthetic irons end up in the liver, are not assimilated and are also very constipating. (See iron).

## Hemorrhaging from the uterus—

Bayberry and Cayenne and get to the hospital. **This is not something to deal with at home. Get help.**

### Constipation—

Lower Bowel Formula        Cascara Sagrada

Much too common during pregnancy. It is important to keep bowels moving not only for basic health reasons, but to also guard against hemorrhoids.

One woman had trouble sleeping and was also constipated. Cascara took care of both problems as Cascara also soothes nerves and promotes sleep.

### False Labor—

Catnip tea, as much as desired or possible.
Blue Cohosh. (See Blue Cohosh)

### Heartburn

| Peppermint Tea | Papaya | Apple Cider Drink |
| Food Enzyme    | Comfrey-Pepsin | Aloe Vera juice |
| Combination    |        |                   |

Choose any of the above and take with meals or as needed. (See apple cider drink-Herbal Recipes and Ailments Chapter.)

### Hemorrhoids and Varicose Veins—(See Ailments)
### Infections, Colds, Etc. during Pregnancy—

Mega Vitamin therapy along with the Infection Fighting herbs have been used safely during pregnancy for the above ailments. (See Acute Illnesses-Ailments Chapter)

### Miscarriage-

1. Catnip and Red Raspberry teas-drink as much as possible.
2. Bayberry and Catnip tea.
3. Lobelia and Cayenne will help relax uterus. Be sure to take Cayenne with Lobelia as it will balance the strong relaxing elements in Lobelia.

Note: One test to determine if fetus is still alive is to take one's temperature first thing in the morning. Have the thermometer by the bed, already shaken down, move as little as possible and take temperature before getting up. It has been found that the fetus is alive if the body temperature is 98.6 or above. (Unless one has chronic low body temperature because of low thyroid metabolism which is unusual during pregnancy.)

**Morning Sickness—**

| | |
|---|---|
| Female Corrective Comb. #1 | Concentrated Alfalfa |
| Red Raspberry tea | 4-5 a day |
| Alfalfa Mint tea | Liver Combination #1 |
| Ginger tea | Green drink or liquid chlorophyll |
| Cloves tea (see recipe)l | B6 with B complex & C |

— Morning sickness is often caused by the hormonal change. Female Corrective combination #1 has been beneficial for this type of morning sickness. Red Raspberry tea alone or a combination with ginger and alfalfa mint has also helped. A combination of the above teas may be used.

— Also nausea can be caused by a congested liver. More and more babies are being born "jaundiced." Yellow bile that is vomited in the morning during the first weeks of pregnancy is often a sign of liver congestion. The liver combinations, or dandelion and yellow dock taken together, have been used for these problems.

— Vitamin B6, taken 200 mg. for 10 days and then 5-9 mg. every day for the rest of the pregnancy, has controlled morning sickness for many women. Taking this with a B Complex vitamin and a C enhances assimilation.

— Cloves tea—(Common cooking spice, use whole cloves) steep 1 tsp. to 1 cup boiling water.

— Nausea in the morning may be caused from low blood sugar, so one may want to keep some teas with honey (Red Raspberry, Peppermint) by the bed.

**Nervousness, Insomnia, Leg Cramps, etc.—**

Nerve and Relaxing Comb. #1 and #3     Calcium Combinations
Teas— Comfrey, Hops, Herbal Sleepy teas
Calcium, at night          B Complex, daytime
The nerve herbs and nerve combinations are very soothing, relaxing and calming to help with the nervous strain of some pregnancies.

**Stretch Marks—**

Good nutrition        B Complex          Vitamin E
Multiple Vitamin      B6 and Zinc
Stretch marks are a deficiency sign of Vitamin B6 and Zinc.

**Toxemia—**

| | | |
|---|---|---|
| B Complex | Vitamin E | Real Food Diet |
| B6 | Vitamin C | Green Drinks |

Exclude all white sugar and white flour products.

**Water Retention (Edema)—**

Kidney/Bladder Combination
Parsley          B Complex, B6 & Vit. C   Eat no salt.
These herbs contain potassium and other minerals so excess water can be reduced safely. Note: Water intake should not be reduced.

**Note: Herbs and juice fasts or mild food diets are safe during pregnancies when problems arise.**


# PREPARING FOR BIRTH

**Delivery—**

Pre-Natal Combination #1 Taken 5 weeks before birth. If any is left over after delivery this combination has also been used to help shrink and tone the uterus after delivery.

Blue Cohosh—used for those who have problems with the cervix dilating. It has been added to the Pre-Natal Combination #1—1 Capsule, 3 times a day for the first 3 weeks; then increased to 2 capsules 3 times a day for the last two weeks or until birth.

2 capsules of Blue Cohosh has also been used to take at the beginning of labor to help cervix dilate.

**Afterpains—**

Nerve & Relaxing Combination #1 (4-6 capsules every two hours has been used.)

| | | |
|---|---|---|
| Capsicum | Wild Lettuce | Valerian Root |
| White Willow | | |


## "AFTER"

**Nursing Mothers**
**To increase milk—**

1. Concentrated Brewer's Yeast—3-4 tablets a day or 16-18 reg-

ular tablets. Start slowly with Brewer's Yeast, it may cause some gas in the beginning.

   2. Concentrated Alfalfa—3-4 capsules a day. Chlorophyll Drink or Green Drink. Make your green drink without Parsley if you are nursing, it is used to dry up milk.

   3. Marshmallow tea—drink warm as often as desired, or 2 capsules 3 or 4 times a day. Other teas Blessed Thistle, Red Raspberry.

   4. Fresh salads, romaine lettuce, sprouts, green drinks, fresh fruits and vegetables, carrot juice, apple juice etc.

**Infected Breast—**

1. Infection Fighting Combinations
2. 1000 mg. Vitamin C every 2 or 3 hours.
3. Treat as for cold. (See Ailments)

**Caked or Infected Breast, Cracked Nipples—**

Vitamin E, Aloe Vera, Comfrey fomentation or poultice.
**To dry up milk—**
Parsley or sage, tea or capsules.

## FOR WOMEN ONLY

## AILMENTS

### Endometriosis, Leucorrhea, Cysts, Tumors, Parasites—

   1. General Cleanser and Parasite Combination #1.
   2. Use Vaginal Bolus Combination (see Other Remedies Women Only)
   3. Lie on a slant board. (An ironing board propped up 12 inches will work) Insert into vagina 2 to 3 ounces mineral water with a small syringe. Retain for 15 to 20 minutes. Expel in toilet. This may need to be done for 10 to 30 days. Cleanses the vaginal tract and uterus.
   4. Infection Fighting Combination #2, especially helpful for Endometriosis and Leucorrhea
   5. Garlic Douche

*Case History:*

   C. used mineral water for 10 days and passed parasites and small round tumor-like tissues from the vaginal tract.

### Estrogen Needs-Hot Flashes

Black Cohosh contains estrogen. (See Black Cohosh and
Menopause)

### Infertility

(See also infertility, Ailments chapter)

Some women have problems conceiving because their bodies are
either too acid or too alkaline. This causes their bodies to kill sperm.
It is possible to be tested for this. A Baking Soda/Honey douche can
be used to correct over-acid problems and a Vinegar douche can be
used for over-alkaline problems. These douches must be used just
prior to intercourse in order to be effective. (See Douches, this
chapter and Body Chemistry in How To Cleanse chapter)

### Menopause

**Herbal Combination—**

1. Calcium Combination #1
2. Female Corrective Combinations, sometimes additional Black
   Cohosh is needed.

**Single Herbs—**

Black Cohosh        Kelp        Sarsaparilla

Black Cohosh contains natural estrogen. Many women find taking
Black Cohosh alone is enough to correct the menopausal symptoms.
Others find it is not enough alone so they take it in combination form
and add an extra Black Cohosh capsule if needed. If you need to
take more than 3 capsules of Black Cohosh a day, you fit in the
category of needing to take a combination plus Black Cohosh.

**Vitamins and Minerals:** Multiple

1. Vitamin E 1000 to 1200 IU.
2. B Complex, with B6 and 250 mg. Pantothenic Acid
3. Vitamin A 50,000 to 75,000 IU.
4. Calcium

### Menstrual Cramping

**Herbs—**

1. Flu Combination #1, excellent results.
2. Ginger tea plus 1 capsule of Black Cohosh has been used.
3. Headache and Pain Combination #1. 4 to 6 capsules
   every 2 hours or as needed has been used.

4. Lobelia and Cayenne. ½ t. of lobelia extract and 2 capsules cayenne every 2 to 4 hours has been used.

**Vitamins—**

Multiple Vitamin and Mineral
B complex and B6
Vitamin C, 1000 to 2000 mg.
Vitamin E, 400 IU
Calcium plus B6, Extra Calcium is needed since calcium is lost through menstrual blood.
**Herbs—** Red Raspberry tea, Ginger, Kelp.
**Diet—** Real Food Diet, green drink or chlorophyll, iron rich foods. (see iron and chlorophyll)
Note: keep colon clean and bowels moving.

### Menstrual Flow, profuse—

1. Bayberry and Cayenne (See Bayberry case history)
2. Catnip tea. As much as desired, flavor with mint tea.
3. Yarrow and Sage. 2 capsules of each daily.
Note: if hemorrhaging, go to the hospital for treatment.

### Ovary, Inflamed

1. Penny Royal 1 or 2 capsules every 3 hours for 4 days.
2. Mineral Water douche
3. Colon cleanse
4. Multiple Vitamin and Mineral
   B Vitamins, B6, and B12
5. Herbs— Cayenne, Lobelia, Chlorophyll
6. Diet— Mild Food Diet, Juice Fast, Real Food Diet.

### Uterus, Cleanse

Juice Fast    Mineral Water Douche    See Endometriosis #3
Note: Many times a liver and/or gall bladder cleanse will also help to cleanse the uterus. An enema is good also. Keeping the colon clean helps the uterus to stay clean.

### Vaginal Discomforts, Itching

1. Mineral Water douche

### Varicose Veins (See Ailments)

### Yeast Infection

1. Garlic douche
2. Comfrey tea or extract douche
3. Acidolphilus Douche or capsule inserted at night

# DOUCHES

**Basic Vinegar**—1 to 2 Tb. White or apple cider vinegar to 1 quart water. (This is good to follow with an Acidophilus douche)

### Other Douches

**Acidolphilus**— open 2 to 4 capsules to 1 quart water. Or you may use watered down yogurt.
**Baking Soda/Honey**— 2 tsp. Baking Soda, 1 tsp. honey to 1 Quart water.
**Cayenne**— ½ tsp. to 1 quart water.
**Cayenne/Vinegar**— ¼ tsp. each to 1 quart water.
**Chlorophyll**— 1 Tb. to 1 quart.
**Comfrey**— use tea or 1-2 Tb. extract per quart.
**Garlic**— 1 or 2 cloves, blend in blender in 1 cup water. Strain, and add enough to make 1 quart.
**Mineral Water**— ¼ to 1/3 cup mineral water to 1 quart water.

### Other Remedies

**Vaginal Bolus**— use Vaginal Bolus Combination or make your own combination with 1 part Goldenseal, 1 part White Oak Bark, ½ part Slippery Elm.

To the powdered herbs—Mix mineral water and olive oil, castor oil, or cocoa butter. Make a firm consistency that can be rolled into tube-like shapes on wax paper. Put in the freezer to firm, let bolus sit at room temperature before using. Insert into vagina at night time, douche the next morning.

# CHAPTER 8

# *Babies*

## BABY NEEDS

### Diet

The first year of nutrition should consist mainly of the mother's breast milk. The beginning breast milk, colostrum, helps to cleanse the baby's system and has many needed nutrients for the newborn. Breast milk is highly nutritious and contains antibodies which give the baby natural immunities to diseases.

Do not buy baby food. It is just as easy to feed the one year old steamed vegetables, (blend in blender) diluted green drink, diluted carrot juice (can mix carrot juice with milk), frozen juice without sugar, mashed bananas, scraped apples, baked potatoes, blended cottage cheese, hard boiled eggs, oatmeal, etc. If additional milk for cereal is needed, raw goat milk has been used. If nursing the baby is not possible and raw or powdered goat milk cannot be found, adding papaya to raw cow's milk helps the baby digest it.

Avoid any foods that contain sugars, white flour, food colorings, or preservatives.

Two excellent books to help you with your baby's diet are *Better Food For Better Babies* by Gena Larson and *Let's Have Healthy Children* by Adele Davis.

**Herbs** work well for babies because:
1. Babies' immune systems haven't been hindered by lots of drugs, so they respond quickly.
2. Herbs have no side effects.

**Vitamins**

Vitamins can be supplied to the baby through the mother's milk which is rich in natural Vitamin A and D.

As the baby gets older a natural chewable or liquid vitamin is good.

**Tips For Babies**

—When giving lemon water or molasses water, etc., to a nursing baby it is better to use a spoon, eye dropper or cup. Nursing babies often get lazy and will not work for mother's milk if they get used to a rubber nipple.

Never allow a baby to drink a bottle while lying on his back or go to sleep and leave a bottle in his mouth. The baby needs to be raised enough so the milk will not slip back into the eustachian tube and cause ear problems. Leaving a bottle in a babe's mouth for them to go to sleep can cause tooth problems.

**Lemon Water—** ½ lemon to 8 ounces of water, add natural sweetener if desired.

**Molasses Water—** ½ to 1 tsp. molasses in water. (See Baby Remedies this chapter)

# HOW TO GIVE HERBS TO BABIES

—Open a capsule, mix with a little water, tea or juice, pour mixture in one side of mouth with spoon, eye dropper, or medicine spoon. Capsules can also be inserted in rectum.

Many times if a nursing baby has a cold, the mother can take the infection fighting combination and vitamins and the baby will get them through the milk.

—Powdered Vitamin C stirred in water or juice has been used.

**How to give a baby an enema**

—Lay baby on his back on towel in tub. Carefully insert lubricated tube into rectum, a little way past anus muscle. Let water (very slowly and without pressure) enter colon—Baby will expel when he feels the need. Repeat as needed until 1 pint has been used. Remember the solution is never given all at once but only the amount that is comfortable, then allow them to expel.

# REMEDIES FOR COMMON BABY PROBLEMS

**Amounts that have been used for baby for infections, colds, flu, etc.**

1 capsule infection fighting combination, 3 or 4 times a day until symptoms disappear. 1 capsule of a specific ailment combination (Lung, Kidney/Bladder etc.) may be added to it if the baby has other symptoms. (cough or kidney infection etc.)

**Colds and Acute Illnesses—**

1. Infection Fighting Combinations plus ⅛ to ¼ tsp. Garlic extract.(Adding garlic to these combinations speeds healing. Because garlic extract is liquid it is one of the easiest and best methods to use for infection in babies. An odorless garlic extract is available.)
2. 1 capsule Herbal Combination specific to ailment (cough, eye infection, etc.)
3. 500—1000 mg. Vitamin C. every 2 or 3 hours.
4. Broths, soups, steamed vegetables, juices, etc.
5. Cleanse colon with enema, or by giving ⅛ to ¼ capsule Cascara in juice or water, prune juice, or molasses water.

**Colic—Hiccups—**

1. Catnip and Fennel Tincture 3-12 drops depending on age has been used. (3-4 for newborn and work up, see Stomach ache, Ailments chapter.) Drops can be put in a teaspoon with warm water or in a bottle. Catnip/Fennel Bottle—use warm water, add tincture and tiny amount of honey or molasses. This bottle can be taken with you in case of colic, or hiccups away from home.
2. Catnip and Peppermint Tea.

**Constipation—**

1. Molasses water
2. Licorice Tea
3. Diluted prune juice.
4. Pears and prunes
5. ¼ capsule Cascara

**Coughs—** treat as for colds

1. Peppermint and Red Raspberry tea with lemon and a little pure maple syrup.

2. Lung combinations and Infection Fighting Combinations
3. Lemon water
4. Mustard plaster or Onion pack if chest is congested. (See Herbal Recipes)

**Cradle Cap—**

Gently, but firmly and thoroughly wash scalp daily with wash cloth and plain water to prevent cradle cap. If problem should arise aloe vera shampoo has been used.

**Croup—** Treat as cold

1. Lobelia extract—2 to 5 drops (not more than 10) on tongue will relax muscles in throat.
2. Infection Fighting Combination and Lung Combination
3. Eucalyptus oil in steamer.
4. Eucalyptus salve or ointment rubbed on chest and neck.

**Diaper Rash—**

1. Aloe Vera Gel
2. Cornstarch
3. Mineral Water-helps sore bottom
4. Creams containing zinc
5. See yeast infection

**Diarrhea—**

1. **Slippery Elm Mixture:** 1T. Slippery Elm to 1 pint cooled scalded skim milk. Feed 1 to 2 T of mixture each time there is an elimination. Liquid intake for baby is important when using Slippery Elm.
2. **Slippery Elm Pudding:** 1-1½ tsp. Slippery Elm and a tiny amount of molasses, mixed with enough water to make it pudding consistency. No cooking necessary, feed as is to the baby. Most babies will eat this, tastes somewhat like burnt caramel.
3. 1 tsp. of whole cloves steeped in 1 quart water—strain—let baby drink as much as he wants, helps with cramping and liquid intake.
4. Oatmeal water—put twice or three times the amount of water over rolled oats. Cook as directed for oatmeal—but just use the water until symptoms are relieved—then start using the oatmeal.
5. Mashed banana, scraped apple, Carob milk.
6. Acidophilus—Important to restore friendly bacteria to intestines.

NOTE: **If baby's bottom is inflamed** then the colon will also be inflamed. A Slippery Elm enema is a quick way to soothe, heal, and coat the lining of the colon. Blend 1 tsp. Slippery Elm to 1 pint water.

### Case History

A baby had diarrhea that had lasted two weeks. He was fed one tablespoon of Slippery Elm mixture every hour or every time there was an elimination. In just a few hours the diarrhea was completely gone. The stools were normal by the next day.

**Earache**— See earache in Ailments

**Eyes**— infected or clogged eye duct.
Make tea of eyewash combinaton, strain and drop into eye with eyedropper. (See Case History under Eyewash Combination)

### Fever—

1. Combination of Peppermint, Red Raspberry and Catnip tea.
2. Tepid bath of Vinegar and Salt or Ginger (see Herbal Recipes)
3. Catnip tea enema, 2 t. Catnip to 1 pint water-steep and cool.
**An enema usually will bring a fever down immediately.**
NOTE: Check temperature frequently with thermometer, feeling the skin is not adequate.
(See Case History under Peppermint)

### Jaundice—

1. Prick a 100 IU of Vitamin E and squirt in mouth. Usually only takes one capsule before jaundice symptoms disappear. Occasionally another capsule taken 12 hours later may be necessary.
2. Lemon water helps to cleanse liver. Add a little molasses or *pure* maple syrup to sweeten.
3. Potato pack on liver. Blend potato in small amount of distilled water so it is still thick or grate potato. Apply to liver area as a poultice. Change poultice in two hours. This will help to cleanse liver very safely and quickly.
4. Garlic enema. If jaundice does not clear up in 24 to 36 hours

or the count starts getting higher. 1 clove garlic to 1 pint water blend—strain.

### Restlessness—

1. A warm water bath is calming
2. ¼ to ½ tsp. Lobelia tincture rubbed on shoulders.
3. Chamomile, Comfrey tea.

### Sore gums—

Swab gums with mineral water, aloe vera gel or juice, or goldenseal tea using a cotton swab or cottonball.

**Sore Throat**—Treat as a cold (See Colds and Acute Illnesses in this chapter)

Give 1 to 3 Tb. pineapple juice several times throughout the day. Pineapple juice has the ability to kill some viruses.

### Stuffy nose—

1. Dissolve ½ tsp. salt in 1 C. warm water. Put 2 drops of solution in each nostril. Wait 45 minutes then suction out mucus with small nose syringe.
2. Goldenseal tea, strained can be used as a nose drop.

**Teething**—Rub a little lobelia extract on gums.

**Tonsillitis**— Treat as a Cold (see colds and acute illnesses this chapter)

1. Infection Fighting Combination #1.

### Yeast Infection—

1. Apply garlic water to baby's bottom.
2. Garlic by mouth. Use garlic extract or prick garlic oil capsule and squirt in mouth.
3. Garlic enema to clear out the colon. Apply Mineral Water, garlic extract, or garlic water to sore bottom.
4. Acidolphilus, by mouth, or capsule can be inserted in rectum.

# CHILDHOOD DISEASES

**To help prevent contagious diseases after exposure—**

1 capsule cayenne 3 times a day and take extra C, 1000 mg. or more daily for 3 or 4 days. Dandelion is also a disease preventative (See Hepatitis, Ailments Chapter). Herbal laxatives also help toxins to be eliminated.

**If a contagious disease does develop, symptoms can be minimized by treating as a cold. (See Cold or Acute Illnesses this chapter)**

**Chicken Pox**

1.  Baths, tepid water-Peppermint, ginger, or vinegar/salt.
2.  Topically-Aloe Vera juice or gel, comfrey extract to pox.
3.  Orally-⅛ to ¼ t. Lobelia and 1 Cayenne capsule or tincture of Cayenne every 3 or 4 hours. Also 1000 mg. Vitamin C every 2 or 3 hours.
4.  If child is **not** running a fever—put child under heat lamp for few minutes after bath, it helps dry up pox. **Note: do not leave child unattended.**

**Mumps**—Treat as an acute illness (See colds and Acute Illness this chapter)

1.  Apply topically to swollen glands
    a.  Onion pack
    b.  Mullein pack (1 T. Mullein, 1 T lobelia powder, 1½ Slippery Elm, mix with mineral water.)
2.  Infection Fighting Comb #2—2 capsules every 3 or 4 hours has been used and ¼ to ½ t. Lobelia. Helps to alleviate symptoms in gland.
4.  Baths—relaxing, releases toxins through skin.
    Ginger or Vinegar/Salt Baths (see Herbal Recipes)
5.  Diet—light. Juices, soups, etc.

**Measles**—Treat as a cold or acute illness
(See Colds and Accute Illness this chapter)

1.  Use baths and instructions of other childhood diseases.
2.  Catnip—Peppermint tea—drink freely

CHAPTER **9**

# Ailments and Remedies

## AILMENTS

The theory of using herbs and vitamin therapy for illness is basically the same for each ailment:
1. Help the body to eliminate the illness by cleansing colon with herbal laxatives, enemas and/or colonics.
2. Take the herbs for specific ailment and those that help move toxins into eliminating organs.
3. Take mega doses of vitamins specific to the ailment to give the body strength.
4. Keep diet light so the body can use energy to fight illness instead of heavy digestion.

### Basic Instructions for Vitamins and Minerals

Foundation: Natural Multiple Vitamin & Mineral Supplement.

#### Mega—Therapy

#### Adults

Vitamin A—75,000-100,000 IU/day for 5 days, then skip a day.
Vitamin C—1,000 mg. every hour. After second day take with calcium and B complex, so C won't act as a chelating agent.
Vitamin E— 400 to 800 IU daily.

Follow the same instructions with these decreased amounts for the ages listed below. For questions See Vitamin Chapter.

|            | 12 to adult   | 6 to 12       | 3 to 6          |
|------------|---------------|---------------|-----------------|
| Vitamin A— | 75,000/day    | 25-50,000/day | 10-20,000/day   |
| Vitamin C— | same as adult | same as adult | same as adult   |
| Vitamin E— | 200 IU/day    | 100 IU/day    | multiple enough |

## Food for Acute Illness

1. Peppermint tea, Chamomile, alfalfa-mint, Red Raspberry, and other tonic teas.
2. Vegetable juices.
3. Vegetable broths or soup
   a. carrots, onions, parsley, potato, etc.
   b. potato-onion soup (red potatoe, including skins)
   c. chicken soup (remove skins before cooking.)
4. Small quantities of fruit juice; two 4 ounce servings per day maximum (no citrus juices, except lemon.)
5. Steamed vegetables
6. Baked potato
7. Yogurt—Cottage Cheese
8. Back to Mild Food Diet.
9. Back to Real Food Diet.
   *No sugar, breads, meat, or junk food during acute illness.

### Exercise during Acute Illness

When someone is very ill, walking may be all that is possible and even short walks may require the aid of another person. Walking barefoot on the grass has been known to help one's energy level.

\*\*\*\*\*\*\*\*\*\*\*\*\*\*

## Basic instructions for illness

### Acute Illness and Colds

1. Use an Herbal Infection Fighting Combination plus garlic. (Adding garlic to these combinations speeds healing.) We use these amounts for Adults: 4 capsules 3 or 4 times a day; Ages 12-18:3 capsules 3 or 4 times a day; Ages 6-12:2 capsules 3 or 4 times a day; Ages baby to 6: 1 capsule 3 or 4 times a day.
2. 1-2 capsules Herbal Combination specific to ailment (cough, kidney, etc.) may be added to the Infection Fighting Combinations. (For example for adults with a cold and cough we would take 4 capsules of an Infection Fighting Combinaton and 1-2 capsules of a Lung Combination every 3 or 4 hours.)
3. Multiple Vitamin and Mineral Supplement plus B Complex.
4. Vitamin A—50,000 to 100,000 IU a day (adults) for 5 days. Then skip a day.
5. Vitamin C—1,000 mg. every 2 or 3 hours. Add calcium and B Complex after second day.
6. Cleanse colon with herbal laxatives, enemas, and/or colonics.

\*\*\*\*\*\*\*\*\*\*\*\*\*\*

# ACNE

Sometimes caused by hormonal imbalances, otherwise caused when body needs to be cleansed.

**Herbal Combinations:**

Blood Purifier Combinations  
Female Corrective Combinations  
   balances female hormones  

Prostate Combinations  
   balances male hormones  
Allergy Combination #1k  
   helps in some cases  

**Single Herbs:**

| | | |
|---|---|---|
| Alfalfa | Chickweed | **Redmond Clay** |
| **Aloe Vera** | **Dandelion** | Sarsaparilla |
| **Burdock** | **Echinacea** | Valerian |
| Cascara Sagrada | **Ginseng** | **Yellow Dock** |
| Cayenne | **Kelp** | |
| **Chaparral** | **Red Clover** | |

Opening an aloe leaf or using gel on blemishes helps clear up skin. Aloe Vera skin care products and herbal masques are available. A Chaparral Scrub may be used (see remedies). Redmond Clay on a blemish can bring it to a head in several hours (see Redmond Clay).

**Vitamins and Minerals:** Natural Multiple Vit. & Min. Supplement Mega-Therapy of A, C, E., B Complex, Vitamin D & F, Zinc, Sulfur.
**Diet:** Real Food Diet, Juice fasts, Green Drink or chlorophyll, No sugar, chocolate, soda pop, etc. Reduce fat in diet.
**Other-**Catnip/Garlic Enemas.

# ALLERGIES

Many allergies clear up when body chemistry is balanced, when body is given nutrients to fight allergies, and when natural antihistamines are used.
**Herbal Combinations:**
Allergy Combination #1       Lung Combinations
Eye Wash Combination #1      Chinese Herbal Oils

**Single Herbs:**

| | | |
|---|---|---|
| Alfalfa | **Comfrey** | **Lobelia** |
| Aloe Vera | **Eyebright** | Marshmallow |
| Black Cohosh | Fenugreek | Papaya |
| Burdock | **Garlic** | Parsley |
| Chaparral | Goldenseal | |
| Chickweed | Juniper Berries | |

**Vitamins & Minerals:** Natural Multiple Vit. & Min. Supplement B Complex, Mega—Vitamin Therapy A, C., **Pantothenic Acid** 100 mg. 3 times a day.
**Diet:** Real Food Diet, Juice Fasts, Mild Food Diet, Green Drinks or chlorophyll, Bee Pollen (start with small amounts. See Bee Pollen.)
**Other—**Catnip/Garlic Enemas.

# ALCOHOLISM

**Herbal Combinations:**
Nerve & Relaxing Combinations #1, #2, #3 or 4
**Single Herbs:**

| Cayenne | Passion Flower | Scullcap |
|---|---|---|

**Vitamins & Minerals:** Natural Multiple Vit. & Min. Supplement
B Complex, B6, Pangamic Acid (B15), Magnesium, Mega A, C, E,.
**Diet:** Real Food Diet, A Juice Fast is a good way to start for this
ailment; then go to Mild Food Diet.

# ANEMIA

**Herbal Combinations:**
Blood Builder Combinaton #1 and #2
**Single Herbs:**

| Alfalfa | Dandelion | Kelp |
|---|---|---|
| Barberry | Fenugreek | Thyme |
| Comfrey | Garlic | Yellow Dock |

Note: Most anemic problems clear up when dandelion is taken. It
restores the nutrient salts. Anemia is almost always caused by
deficiency of these nutritive salts. (See Dandelion)
**Vitamins & Minerals:** Natural Multiple Vit. & Min. Supplement B
Complex, B12, E, C aids iron assimilation, **Calcium, Natural Che-
lated iron Supplement.**
**Diet:** Real Food Diet, Green Drink or **Chlorophyll,** Bee Pollen,
Beets and Beet juice, Black Cherries, Molasses, Bananas, Apricots,
Wheat Grass, Barley Green, Spirulina. (See Iron)

# ARTERIOSCLERIOSIS—ATHEROSCLEROSIS
### (Hardening of Arteries—Plaquing of arteries)

**Herbal Combinations:**

Blood Pressure & Heart Combinations
Blood Purifying Combinations

**Single Herbs:**

| | | |
|---|---|---|
| Aloe Vera Juice | **Garlic** | **Hawthorne** |
| **Cayenne** | Golden Seal | Rose Hips |
| Comfrey | Kelp | Taheebo |

**Vitamins & Minerals:** Natural Multiple Vit. & Min. Supplement

B Complex, B6, **Rutin (Bioflavoids),** Mega—A, C, E, **Lecithin, Choline, Inositol,** Calcium, Chromium, Magnesium.

Some believe Atherosclerosis to be a deficiency disease of Vitamin C.

**Diet:** Real Food Diet, Juice Fasts, Mild Food Diet, **Raw Foods, Green Drinks** or **Chlorophyll** Drink, Apple Cider Vinegar.

(See also Heart)

# ARTHRITIS

**Herbal Combinations:**

| | |
|---|---|
| Headache & Pain Comb. #1 | Chines Herbal Oils, |
| Arthritis Combinations | rub on painful areas |

**Single Herbs:**

| | | |
|---|---|---|
| **Alfalfa** | **Comfrey** | Parsley |
| **Aloe Vera** | Fenugreek | Safflower |
| Black Cohosh | Garlic | **Valerian Root** |
| Blessed Thistle | Juniper Berries | **White Willow** |
| **Burdock** | **Kelp** | use for aspirin |
| **Cayenne** | Licorice Root | Yarrow |
| **Chaparral** | Lobelia | |

**Vitamins & Minerals:** Natural Multiple Vit. & Min. Supplement,

Pantothenic Acid, Mega—A, C, E., Calcium, Potassium, Brewer's Yeast.

**Diet:** Real Food Diet, Mild Food Diet, Juice Fasts, mostly vegetarian diet, green drink, carrot juice.

No red meat, sugars, or refined foods.

## Arthritis Drink

2 cups water (distilled, purified, or mineral water.)

1 large apple—wash, scrub to take off wax and poisons.
2 lemons— wash, scrub to take off wax and poisons.
Cut up apple and lemons, and blend in blender with water. Put 3 Tb. blended mixture in pineapple, apple, or orange juice and drink. This can be drunk once a day or more often if desired. It has helped increase mobility and decrease pain when used regularly.

# ASTHMA

## Herbal Combinations

Allergy Combination #1       Tincture of Lobelia for
Lung Combinations               acute attack

## Single Herbs:

| | | |
|---|---|---|
| **Alfalfa** | Ginseng | Saw Palmetto |
| Black Cohosh | Goldenseal | Slippery Elm |
| **Cayenne** | Licorice Root | Taheebo |
| Chamomile | **Lobelia** | Thyme |
| **Comfrey** | Marshmallow | Valerian |
| **Fenugreek** | **Mullein** | White Willow |
| **Garlic** | **Myrrh** | Wood Betony |
| Ginger | Parsley | |

**Vitamins & Minerals:** Natural Multiple Vit. & Min. Supplement

B Complex, Mega A, C, E, Pantothenic Acid 100 mg. 3 times a day, Calcium, Magnesium, Potassium, Manganese, Bee Pollen—start with small amounts.
**Diet:** Real Food Diet, **Juice Fasts,** Mild Food Diet, mostly fresh juices, raw vegetables, green drink. Vegetarian diet. Apple Cider Vinegar.

No mucous forming foods, milk, meat, breads, sugars. Reduce fat intake.
**Other—**
Colon Cleanses, Catnip/Garlic Enemas, Colonics. Onion Poultice on chest.

# ATHLETE'S FOOT

Apply Black Walnut Tincture

# BALDNESS

**Herbal Combinations:**

Combination Hair, Skin and Nails #1

**Single Herbs:**

Aloe Vera shampoos    Jojoba                    Taheebo

**Vitamins & Minerals:** Natural Multiple Vit. & Min. Supplement

B Vitamins, Pantothenic Acid, Biotin, Zinc.
**Diet:** Real Food Diet, Juice Fasts, Green Drink.
**Other—**Bring Circulation to head area, massage, use slant board.

# BED WETTING

—Kidney/Bladder Combination #1, one hour before bedtime.
—Cornsilk tea—take cornsilk off corn cob, steep and strain. Give 1 hour before bedtime.
—Sometimes eating a food the person is allergic to will cause bed wetting. If other methods don't work check out possible allergy problems. See also Kidneys.
—Compressed nerve—See chiropractor.

**Single Herbs—**
**Cornsilk**            **Marshmallow**        **Uva Ursi**
**Juniper Berries**     **Parsley**

# BEE & WASP STINGS, SPIDER & MOSQUITO BITES

**Emergency treatment for allergic reactions:**
1.  Blue Cohosh or Black Cohosh poultice on area. (Open Capsule and mix with a little water and apply to area. Repeat in 5 or 10 minutes.)
2.  One tsp, 2 capsules, or ¼ tsp tincture of Cayenne in warm water. Take orally.
3.  Massive doses of Vitamin C.
4.  Massive doses of Calcium
5.  Tobacco poultices work also.

### Bee & Wasp Stings

Take 4 capsules Infection fighting Combination 3 times a day and 1000 mg. Vitamin C every hour. Choose the following as needed.

—Stinger needs to be removed before it can heal. Carefully remove stinger, do not squeeze it and allow more poison in. Redmond Clay or honey will pull out stinger. Wet clay with a little water and apply to sting.

—Apply ice for pain and swelling.

—Apply mineral water, then Poultice Comb. #1 mixed with mineral water to pull poison.

—Plantain, Charcoal, Blessed Thistle, Chamomile poultices

### Mosquito & Spider Bites

For poisonous bites or severe reactions see instructions under Bee and Wasp Stings.

For relief of itching and swelling:

—Comfrey extract, Aloe Vera, Eucalyptus Oil, Chinese Herbal Oils, or Lemon Juice.

**For prevention:**

1. Take a multiple and a B complex daily.
2. Eat raw onion.

## BLEEDING/HEMORRHAGING

Apply Cayenne to wound and take 2 capsules by mouth with warm water.

**Bleeding in the mouth**—Chew poked Vitamin E capsule.

**From uterus**—take 2 capsules Cayenne and add 2 capsules Bayberry with warm water and **go to the hospital.**

## BLOOD POISONING

Treat as cold, See also Gangrene

# BLOOD PRESSURE

## High Blood Pressure
## Herbal Combinations

Blood Pressure Combinations       Nerve & Relaxing Combinations

### Single Herbs:

| | | |
|---|---|---|
| **Aloe Vera** | **Cayenne** | Hops |
| Black Cohosh | **Garlic** | Kelp |
| Blue Cohosh | Gotu Kola | Scullcap |
| Cascara Sagrada | **Hawthorne** | Valerian Root |

**Vitamins & Minerals:** Natural Multiple Vit. & Min. Supplement

B Complex, Rutin, Mega A, C, E. Note: Start with 100 IU/day of E and work up gradually over a period of weeks to 400 to 600 IU/day. (See Vitamin E toxicity section)
**Diet:** Real Food Diet, Juice fasts, Mild Food Diet, Green Drink or Chlorophyll, Wheat Grass, Barley Green Bee Pollen.
**Other:** Garlic enemas.

### Low Blood Pressure

Follow as if for High Blood Pressure, these herbs are excellent for Low Blood Pressure.

### Single Herbs:

| | | |
|---|---|---|
| **Cayenne** | **Hawthorne** | Valerian Root |
| **Dandelion** | **Kelp** | Yarrow |
| **Garlic** | Parsley | Yellow Dock |
| Ginger | Peppermint | |

# BOILS

Packs made from Comfrey, Goldenseal, Slippery Elm mixed with mineral water will pull. Poultice Combination #1, Clay packs also help.

# BRONCHITIS

## Herbal Combinations:

Lung Combinations                    Infection Fighting Combination
                                          plus Garlic

## Single Herbs:

| | | |
|---|---|---|
| Bayberry | **Garlic** | Red Clover |
| Black Cohosh | **Ginger** | Red Raspberry |
| Blue Cohosh | **Goldenseal** | Sage |
| Camomile | Hops | Saw Palmetto |
| Catnip | Licorice root | Slippery Elm |
| **Cayenne** | **Lobelia** | Taheebo |
| Chickweed | Marshmallow | Uva Ursi |
| **Comfrey** | **Mullein** | Valerian Root |
| Dandelion | **Myrrh** | **Yarrow** |
| **Echinacea** | Peach Bark | Yellow Dock |
| Fennel | **Peppermint** | |
| **Fenugreek** | **Poke Root** | |

**Vitamins & Minerals:** Natural Multiple Vit. & Min. Supplement
   B Complex, Mega A, C, E, treat as for cold.
**Diet:** Real Food Diet, Soups, Broths, Mild Food Diet, Green Drink.
**Other—**Mustard Plaster or onion pack to chest area (See Herbal Recipes)
   —Catnip/Garlic enemas daily.
   —Eucalyptus or Apple Cider Vinegar in steamer.

# BRUISES—See also wounds

   —Apply onion or comfrey poultice
   —Take Poultice Combination and Vitamin E internally.
   —Apply Chinese Herbal Oils

# BURNS

## For minor Burns:

1st Degree: Reddened Skin.
1. Use ice on burn until pain is gone.
2. Open fresh aloe vera leaf or use aloe vera salve.
3. Chinese Herbal Oils.
4. Redmond Clay pack.

## For serious burns:

2nd Degree: Reddened skin and blisters.
3rd Degree: Skin destroyed and charred.
1. Treat for shock. Cayenne—¼ tsp. tincture, 2 capsules, or 1 tsp in warm water.
2. Cut away loose clothing that is not adhered to the skin. If skin is not charred, can use ice to relieve pain or ice water. If skin is charred—sterile, cold, moist cloths dipped in Aloe Vera Juice or Gel may be used while a poultice is being fixed.
   a. Apply Poultice Combination mixed with Mineral Water (or Aloe Vera Juice or Gel) and Olive Oil (or Vitamin E Oil or Castor Oil) to burn. Before applying poultice gently drop some Vitamin E Oil or Olive Oil on first to prevent pulling when the poultice is removed.
   b. Fresh comfrey leaf poultice (See Herbal Recipes) is soothing to burned area. Apply Vitamin E before using it so it does not stick.
3. Take Infection Fighting Combinations, Poultice Combinations, Pain Combinations, and Vitamin E by mouth.
**Depending on the degree of burn and the percent of the body burned, other medical help may be needed.**

## For Chemical Burns:

Flood with water, some chemical burns can be neutralized with apple cider vinegar. Flood with water again for as long as 20 minutes. Repeat apple cider vinegar if necessary. Apply herbs.

## For grease burns:

Gently remove grease with soap and water. Then treat.
Redmond Clay packs have been used to alleviate pain on grease burns.

## BURSITIS, See Arthritis

## CANKER—COLD SORES

—Take 500 mg. Lysine at first sign. (See Lysine)
—Rinse with mineral water, make tea out of Poultice Combination and rinse mouth; rinse with Goldenseal tea, Aloe Vera juice, or paint with Black Walnut extract.

Rinses can be used every 15 minutes if needed.

For Prevention: take B Complex vitamin, acidophilus, or lysine every day.

## CATARACTS—See Eyes

## CHICKEN POX & CHILDHOOD DISEASES—See Baby Chapter

## CIRCULATION

—Take Cayenne daily, 2 capsules with each meal.
—Take Energy and Fitness Combination #1.
—B Complex, Niacin (See Vitamin B3), Vitamin C and E.
—Exercise
—Clean colon.

## COLDS—See beginning of this chapter.

## COLIC—See Baby Chapter

## COLITIS—See Ulcers

## CONSTIPATION

**Herbal Combinations:**

Lower Bowel Combinations

**Single Herbs:**

| | | |
|---|---|---|
| Alfalfa | Goldenseal | Slippery Elm |
| Burdock | Licorice Root | Turkey Rhubarb |
| **Cascara Sagrada** | Mandrake | Yellow Dock |
| **Chickweed** | Psyllium | |
| Ginger | Raspberry | |

**Vitamins & Minerals:** Natural Multiple Vit. & Min. Supplement, B Complex

**Diet:** Real Food Diet, Juice Fasts, Mild Food Diet, Chlorophyll or Green Drinks, Aloe Vera Juice. Prunes, yogurt, **acidophilus**, whey, brewer's yeast. Eat mostly **whole grains**, **raw vegetables**, **fruits**, **Bran**, Wheat Grass, & Barley Green.

Apple cider drink (1 to 2 tsp cider) to glass first thing in morning and with meals.

**Other:** See enema chapter, for babies see baby chapter.

## CORNS

**Corns:** Apply olive oil to corn, put slice of raw garlic on corn with band aid. This can be done at night time until corn is gone.

## COUGH—See Bronchitis, Cough Syrups, Herbal Recipes

## CRAMPS—See Women Only

## CROUP—See Baby Chapter

## DANDRUFF

Aloe Vera and Jojoba Shampoo, Cleanse system, Juice fasts, A, B Vitamins, Zinc.

## DENTAL CARIES

**Herbal Combinations:**

Calcium Combinations

**Single Herbs:**

| Alfalfa | **Black Walnut** | Kelp |

These herbs contain natural fluoride.

**Vitamins & Minerals:** Natural Multiple Vit. & Min. Supplement B Complex, B6, Vitamin C, Calcium.

**Diet:** Real Food Diet, Juice Fast, Green Drink or chlorophyll, Aloe Vera Juice.

# DIABETES

### Herbal Combinations:

Pancreas Combinations          Nerve & Relaxing Combinations
(See Pancreas Combinations)

### Single Herbs:

| | | |
|---|---|---|
| **Alfalfa** | Dandelion | Marshmallow |
| **Aloe Vera** | **Eyebright** | Safflower |
| Black Cohosh | Fenugreek | Saw Palmetto |
| Blue Cohosh | **Garlic** | Slippery Elm |
| **Cayenne** | **Goldenseal** | **Taheebo** |
| Chickweed | **Juniper Berries** | Yarrow |
| Comfrey | **Kelp** | |

**Vitamins & Minerals:** Natural Multiple Vit. & Min. Supplement **Chromium**, B Complex, B12, B6, Mega A, C, E, Manganese, Sulfur.

**Diet:** Real Food Diet, Green Drinks or Chlorophyll, String beans, Brewer's Yeast, Spirulina, Wheat Grass, Barley Green. Mostly raw foods.

No sugar, white flour products.

**Other:** Exercise is very important, enemas are needed and a positive attitude is mandatory.

# DIARRHEA

Peppermint tea, Cloves tea, Oatmeal water, Slippery Elm, Carob, Acidophilus, Banana.

No wheat products or foods containing fat.

See Diarrhea under Baby Chapter.

# DIGESTION

**Herbal Combinations:**

Digestive Combinations                              Comfrey/Pepsin
(See Digestive Combinations)

**Single Herbs:**

| | | |
|---|---|---|
| **Alfalfa** | Comfrey | Goldenseal |
| **Aloe Vera** | Dandelion | Juniper Berries |
| Barberry | Echinacea | Licorice Root |
| Bayberry | Eyebright | Lobelia |
| Black Cohosh | **Fennel** | Myrrh |
| Blessed Thistle | Fenugreek | **Papaya** |
| Cascara Sagrada | **Garlic** | **Peppermint** |
| **Cayenne** | **Ginger** | |
| **Camomile** | Ginseng | |

**Vitamins & Minerals:** Natural Multiple Vit. & Min. Supplement B Complex, Vitamin F, Magnesium.
**Diet:** Real Food Diet, Juice Fasts, Mild Food Diet, Green Drink or Chlorophyll, Aloe Vera Juice, Apple Cider Vinegar, Bee Pollen, Acidophilus, Wheat Grass, Barley Green, Spirulina.
     Peppermint or Spearmint tea, Camomile or Alfalfa Mint tea, and other tonic teas help digestion. Cider Drink (Sweet and Sour Drink) (See Herbal Recipes)

**Case History:**

   A young man in his 20's was having weight loss and food assimilation problems. He was extremely thin, weak and had no energy. He began taking Digestion Combination #3 every time he ate. He has gained weight and is feeling better than he has ever felt.

# DIVERTICULITIS
## (See Ulcer-Colitis)

# EAR ACHES—Treat as cold

   —Wash out ear with hydrogen peroxide using a small ear syringe. Very gently pulsate peroxide in and out of ear. When bubbling of peroxide diminishes, ear is clean of bacteria. This can be done before adding herbal ear remedies if desired.

—Put 2 or 3 drops of strained onion juice in ear. Grate onion, strain. Then put cotton in ear. Onion juice stops the pain and fights infections. In fact, we have found that onion juice has been the fastest, most effective remedy to stop pain and fight infection.

—2 drops garlic oil, 2 drops lobelia extract. Warm garlic oil in a teaspoon, do not let get too hot. Put warm (body temperature) in ear. Follow the same procedure in heating lobelia and put it in the ear, and place a piece of cotton in the ear.

—Infection Fighting Combination #7 (Extract) can be used as ear drops.

—Ice packs or alternating hot and cold packs help pain. Most people apply heat to earache. Even though this feels good it brings congestion to a small area and is often the cause of broken ear drums.

— Infection fighting combinations by mouth, treat as cold

# ECZEMA

## Herbal Combinations:

Blood Purifier Combinations        Lower Bowel combinations
Hair, Skin, Nails Comb. #1        Infection Fighting Combinations
Calcium Combinations

## Single Herbs:

| | | |
|---|---|---|
| **Aloe Vera** | **Echinacea** | **Redmond Clay** |
| Black Walnut | **Goldenseal** | Slippery Elm |
| **Burdock** | Kelp | Taheebo |
| **Comfrey** | **Myrrh** | White Willow |
| **Dandelion** | Poke Root | |

**Vitamins & Minerals:** Natural Multiple Vit. & Min. Supplement B Complex, Mega A, C, E, D, **Zinc.**
**Diet:** Real Food Diet, Juice Fasts, Mild Food Diet, Green Drink Chlorophyll, Aloe Vera Juice internally and Gel externally, Bee Pollen, Vegetable Diet, mostly raw foods, grains, beans, seeds, Wheat Grass, Barley Green.

No sugars, refined foods, chocolate, meat, or dairy products.
**Other:** Catnip/Garlic Enemas.

## EDEMA OR WATER RETENTION
—Parsley and other diuretic herbs.
—Take 2 capsules of Kidney/Bladder Combinations in morning.
See also Kidney/Bladder or Problems of Pregnancy.

## EMPHYSEMA

**Herbal Combinations:**

Lung Combinations          Infection Fighting Combs. plus garlic.

**Single Herbs:**

| | | |
|---|---|---|
| **Cayenne** | **Garlic** | Myrrh |
| Chickweed | Goldenseal | Rose Hips |
| **Comfrey** | Licorice | Slippery Elm |
| **Echinacea** | **Lobelia** | Thyme |
| **Fenugreek** | Marshmallow | White Oak Bark |
| Fennel | **Mullein** | |

**Vitamins & Minerals:** Natural Multiple Vit. & Min. Supplement B Complex, Pantothenic Acid, Mega A, C, E.
**Diet:** Real Food Diet, Juice Fasts, Mild Food Diet, Chlorophyll, Aloe Vera Juice.
**Other:** Colon cleanse is important. Catnip/Garlic enemas. Exercise: Walking—Deep Breathing exercises.

## EYES—SORE EYES, INFECTED, CATARACTS

**Infected, swollen, inflamed or sore**—make tea of **Eye Wash Combination**, using 1 capsule to ¼ cup boiling water. Cool, strain and use as an eye wash or eye drop. Can be used 3 to 4 times a day as needed. Take infection fighting comb. by mouth 3 to 4 capsules 3 to 4 times a day.
   —Use Aloe vera juice for eye drops. Brings circulation to eye area, healing—use once to twice a day. If Aloe Vera juice has Ascorbic Acid in it, it will sting.

### Cataracts—

**Herbal Combinations:** Eyewash Combination—internally and as drops in eyes 3 times a day. (See Eyewash Combination)
**Single Herbs:** Eyebright 8 to 12 capsules a day. Aloe Vera Juice as eyedrops.

**Eyebright Wash** (Can be stored in refridgerator)

Open 1 capsule eyebright, boil water, steep in 1 ounce water. Strain. Add to 1 ounce of mineral water. Wash eyes twice a day. This can help eye infections also but is especially good for cataracts.

**Vitamins & Minerals:** Natural Multiple Vit. & Min. Supplement B Complex, B2 B6, Choline, Mega A, C, E.
**Diet:** Real Food Diet, Mild Food Diet, Juice Fasts.

For more information: *Better Eyesight Without Glasses*, by Dr. W.H. Bates, and *Cataracts and Glaucoma* by Tobe.
**Other:** Cleanse system with enemas.

## FEMALE PROBLEMS—See For Women Only and Pregnancy Chapter

## FEVER

—Catnip tea enema, cool water to tepid temperature before using. Fever usually persists when colon is congested. A plain enema using plain (tepid) water will also bring down a fever.

—Drink Catnip/Peppermint tea (equal parts mixed) Also Yarrow tea may be added to this mixture.

—Treat as for cold.

—Tepid Ginger bath or tepid vinegar and salt bath. See herbal recipes.

—For child, pour tepid water over shoulders, stomach and back as he sits in tub.

—Cool Water Rub Down—Dip cloth in cool water, squeeze cloth and rub a section of the body keeping the other part of the body lightly covered with sheet. Cover the rubbed section and start on a new section. This brings circulation to surface and cools the body down. Be sure to do face, back of neck, palms, and bottom of the feet.

## FLATULENCE—GAS

—Chlorophyll drinks or Green Drink will neutralize flatuence.

—Peppermint and Spearmint tea will expel gas from colon and stomach. Comfrey, Camomile, and Alfalfa Mint also help.

—Catnip/Fennel Tincture. Can be used often as needed.

—Take Digestive Enzymes with meals.

—See also Digestion.

# FLU-INFLUENZA

—Flu Combination #1. 4 capsules, 3 or 4 times a day for adults, 3 capsules for 12-18, 2 capsules for 6-12 and 1 for 6 and under. (See Flu Combination)

—Aloe Vera Juice, Peppermint, Yarrow, Comfrey, Cloves tea, or Chinese Oils for nausea, fever, stomache pain.

—Enemas (especially when diarrhea is present.)

—Treat as for cold. (See also stomache ache this chapter)

# FOOD POISONINGS

—Eat 1 or 2 heads **iceberg** lettuce.

# GALL BLADDER AND STONES

People who have problems with Gall Bladder and Stones usually eat large amounts of meats and fatty foods. These must be eliminated from the diet, in order to overcome this problem. Going on Juice Fasts, Mild Food Diet and Real Food Diet is strongly recommended.

**Gall Stone Cleanse:**

1. Apple juice fast for 3 days. Take enemas every day.
2. End of 3rd day drink 3 oz. lemon juice mixed with 3 oz olive oil just before going to bed.
3. Sleep on right side with pillow under hip to help concentrate the remedy in the gall bladder area.
4. Take Garlic enema in the morning of the 4th day. Should pass stones. Stones are green and black in color.

—Do not go back to eating normally after a Gall Stone Cleanse, treat this as a Juice Fast and resume eating according to those instructions.

**Case History:**

C. took the 3 day apple juice fast and on the morning of the 4th day when she took the enema she passed 1 cup of gall stones.

# GANGRENE

—Make poultice with Poultice Combination. (See Poultices) Wound may appear worse at first as it pulls toxins out.

—Fomentation of Marshmallow tea (See Fomentations) or plantain poultice.

**Herbal Combinations:**

Poultice Combination, topically
Blood Purifier Combinations, internally

Infection Fighting Combs. plus Garlic, internally

**Single Herbs:**

| | | |
|---|---|---|
| Bayberry | **Chickweed** | **Garlic** |
| Burdock | **Echinacea** | Marshmallow |
| Cayenne | **Plantain** | |

**Vitamins & Minerals:** Natural Multiple Vit. & Min. Supplement Mega Doses A, C, E. Treat as cold.
**Diet:** Real Food Diet, Juice Fast, Green Drink.
**Other:** Enemas—Garlic/Catnip daily.

# GOUT

Gout usually goes hand in hand with Arthritis. Wrong eating habits and poor diet are the major causes of it, especially too much eating of red meat. See Arthritis.

# HALITOSIS—(Bad Breath)

Usually caused from sluggish intestinal system and chronic constipation. Can also happen when the body is cleansing.

**Single Herbs:**

| | | |
|---|---|---|
| Alfalfa | Barberry | Peppermint |

**Vitamins & Minerals:** Natural Multiple Vit. & Min. Supplement B Complex.
**Diet:** Real Food Diet, Juice Fasts, Mild Food Diet, Green Drink or Chlorophyll.

**Other:** Cleanse colon, garlic/catnip enemas.

# HAY FEVER—See Asthma

# HEADACHE & MIGRAINE HEADACHE

Headaches are caused by many reasons: Hypoglycemia, congested colon, stress, spinal maladjustment, illness, mineral or vitamin deficiencies, hormonal imbalances, etc. Many times when you treat a headache you are treating the symptom and not the cause. Try to find out what is causing the headache and then remove the cause.
   —Headache and Pain Combinations
   —Chinese Herbal Oils—topically rubbed on head, temple.
   —Stress or Nerve Combinations
   —B Vitamins and Calcium.

## Migraine Headaches and Cluster Headaches:

   —Headache Combination #1. This combination contains Fenugreek and Thyme which help vascular headaches.
   People who suffer from migraine headaches are notorious for their poor eating habits. Elimination of sugar, chocolate, refined foods are a must.
   —Some people have found that taking B Vitamins daily prevents them from getting headaches.
   — Chiropractic care has worked wonders for Migraine and other headaches.

# HEART

## Herbal Combinations:

Blood Pressure and Heart Combinations
Nerve and Relaxing Combinations
Calcium Combinations

## Single Herbs:

| | | |
|---|---|---|
| Barberry | **Cayenne** | **Garlic** |
| Black Cohosh | Blessed Thistle | Goldenseal |

| | | |
|---|---|---|
| Gotu Kola | **Licorice** | Scullcap |
| **Hawthorne** | **Lobelia** | **Valerian Root** |
| Juniper Berries | **Peppermint** | Wood Betony |
| **Kelp** | Sage | |

## For Heart Palpitations:

Hawthorne, Peppermint, Sage, Valerian Root, Mineral Water.

Note: ½ cup Mineral Water has been used after a heart attack to regulate heart beat. For palpitations ¼ cup has been used. Minerals help regulate the heart.

**Vitamins & Minerals:** Natural Multiple Vit. & Min. Supplement, B Complex, B6, Mega A, C. Vitamin E start with 100 IU and work up (see Vitamin E) The amount of Vitamin E should be individually determined for each person. Vitamin E is not toxic, but makes the heart more efficient so amounts must be worked up slowly.

Calcium, Magnesium, Selenium, Chromium, **Potassium**, Choline-(Lecithin), Bee Pollen, Mineral Water.

**Diet:** Real Food Diet, Juice Fasts, Mild Food Diet, Green Drink or Chlorophyll. Juice fasts help prevent thrombosis and stroke.

No refined foods, alcohol, coffee, sugar, salt, or red meat.

# HEARTBURN

—1 tsp apple cider vinegar in ½ cup warm water. Drink as needed.

—15 to 20 drops Catnip/Fennel tincture in warm water. Helps pain and aids digestion. Can be repeated as needed.

—Digestive food enzymes containing several enzymes.

—Peppermint tea, Aloe Vera juice.

(See Cider Drink, p.236.)

# HEMORRHOIDS

**Herbal Combinations:**

Lower Bowel Combination

**Single Herbs:**

| | | |
|---|---|---|
| **Cascara Sagrada** | **Goldenseal** | **White Oak Bark** |
| **Collinsonia** | Slippery Elm | Yarrow |

**Vitamins & Minerals:** Natural Multiple Vit. & Min. Supplement
   Vitamin A, **C**—2000-3000 mg./day, **E**—600-800 IU, **B Complex**,
Rutin, B6.
**Diet:** Real Food Diet, Same as for constipation. Bee Pollen. Drink
plenty of liquids.
   No refined foods, sugar.

### White Oak Bark/Goldenseal Retention Enema
(For Hemorrhoids)

   This enema is a retention enema. Which means you retain a small
amount of the mixture in the colon overnight.

Why—    Used to reduce swelling fight infection and relieve pain of
        hemorrhoids and bleeding hemorrhoids. Takes soreness
        out of area, White Oak Bark also acts as an astringent to
        shrink hemorrhoids.

How—    Pour 1 cup boiling water over 2 tsp. powdered White Oak
        Bark, and 2 tsp powdered Goldenseal, let steep. Strain and
        cool. Insert 1 or 2 ounces and retain overnight for internal
        hemorrhoids. Lay a poultice or pack of tea on external
        hemorrhoids.

   Also Goldenseal/White Oak Bark, Slippery Elm, or Yarrow
fomentations can be used on external hemorrhoids.

# HERPES

   —Black Walnut Extract, apply to area.
   —Aloe Vera Gel, apply to area, drink juice.
   —Lysine.
   —Comfrey extract, prick blisters and apply to area several times
a day.

# HEPATITIS
(See also Liver)

**Herbal Combinations:**

Liver/Gall Combinations       Dandelion and Yellow Dock taken to-
                              gether

**Single Herbs:**

| | | |
|---|---|---|
| Cayenne | Lobelia | **Yellow Dock** |
| **Dandelion** | Yarrow | |

**Vitamins & Minerals:** Natural Multiple  Vit. & Min. Supplement
**Vitamin C.** See *Dr. Wright's Book of Nutritional Therapy* for excellent information on using Vitamin C with Hepatitis. If large doses of Vitamin C are used, give B Complex and Calcium to prevent C from washing them out. B Complex, Mega A, and E. All Minerals.
**Diet:** Real Food Diet, Mild Food Diet, Juice Fasts, Green Drink.
   —Very important to have a low fat diet. The liver cannot handle fats during hepatitis.
**Other:** Catnip/Garlic enemas.

**Case History:**

   P., a four-year-old child was exposed to hepatitis and came down with the disease. His Hepatitis blood tests were extremely high. The doctor said it was one of the worst cases of hepatitis he had seen in a young child for years. The suggested treatment was good food and bed rest to allow the body to heal itself. P.'s parents gave 4 capsules Dandelion, and 4 capsules Yellow Dock a day. They also gave 1 capsule of Liver Combination #1 once a day. In 9 days, the child's count was back to almost normal.
   For an adult they would have given 8 capsules of Dandelion and Yellow Dock each a day. The rest of the family took a preventative dose of Dandelion and Yellow Dock, which was ½ the regular dose. No one else came down with Hepatitis.

## HIATAL HERNIA

   —Drink Poultice Combination (Slippery Elm can be added) stirred in water to coat entire esophagal tract including hernia and relieve symptoms. Capsules will not work here.
   —Mineral water, drink 1-2 ounces 2 or 3 times a day.
   —Aloe Vera Juice 1 or 2 ounces 2 times a day.
   Mineral water and Aloe Vera juice can be alternated.
   (See also Slippery Elm.)

## HIGH BLOOD PRESSURE-HYPERTENSION See Blood Pressure

# HOARSENESS-LARYNGITIS

—1 tsp of cider vinegar to half glass water every hour.
—Drink Licorice Root mixed with water. See Licorice Root Case History.
—Treat as cold.

## Herbal Combinations:

Infection Fighting Combination plus Garlic

## Single Herbs:

| | | |
|---|---|---|
| **Aloe Vera** | Goldenseal | Sage |
| Chickweed | **Licorice Root** | Slippery Elm |
| Comfrey | Lobelia | |
| Fennel | Marshmallow | |

## Vitamins & Minerals

Natural Multiple Vit. & Min. Supplement B Complex, Pantothenic Acid, Mega A, C, E.—Treat as cold.
**Diet:** Real Food Diet, Juice Fasts, Mild Food Diet, Chlorophyll, Lemon Juice, Apple cider Vinegar.

# HORMONE IMBALANCE

## Herbal Combinations:

Female Corrective Combinations for women (See Women Only) Prostate Combinations for men.

## Single Herbs:

| | | |
|---|---|---|
| **Bayberry** | **Ginseng** | **Sarsaparilla** |
| **Black Cohosh** | Ho Sho Wu | **Sage** |
| **Blessed Thistle** | **Kelp** | Saw Palmetto |
| Camomile | Licorice Root | **Yarrow** |
| **Damiana** | **Red Raspberry** | |

Note: Applied Kinesiology (Muscle Response Testing) often helps to find which hormonal herbs are specific to individual.
**Vitamins & Minerals:** Natural Multiple Vit. & Min. Supplement B Complex

**Diet:** Real Food Diet, Juice Fasts, Mild Food Diet, Green Drinks or Chlorophyll, Bee Pollen.

## HOT FLASHES (See For Women Only)

## HYPERACTIVE—HYPERKINETIC CHILDREN

**Herbal Combinations:**

Nerve Combinations                Calcium Combinations

**Single Herbs:**

| Camomile | **Lobelia** | Thyme |
| Catnip | **Passion Flower** | **Valerian Root** |
| **Hops** | **Scullcap** | **Wood Betony** |

**Vitamins & Minerals:** Natural Multiple Vit. & Min. Supplement
   It is possible to get Natural Vitamins in either chewable or in liquid form so even babies and small children can take them. B Complex is very important. Mega A, C, E. All minerals, especially magnesium and calcium.

**Diet:** Real Food Diet, **Feingold Diet,** Mild Food Diet, Juice Fasts, Chlorophyll or Green Drink, Bee Pollen.
   **No preservatives, artificial colorings or flavorings, no sugar.**

## HYPOGLYCEMIA

(See also Pancreas Combinations in Combination Chapter)

**Herbal Combinations:**

Pancreas Combinations              Blood Builder Combinations

**Single Herbs:**

| Alfalfa | **Dandelion** | **Licorice Root** |
| **Cayenne** | Kelp | **Safflower** |
| Comfrey | **Hawthorne** | |

   Safflower helps hypoglycemics with muscle aches and fatigue when they exercise.

**Vitamins & Minerals:** Natural Multiple Vit. & Min. Supplement
   **B Complex,** B6, Pantothenic Acid, Mega A, C, E, Zinc,
**Chromium**.
**Diet:** Real Food Diet, Juice Fasts—mostly vegetable, Mild Food Diet,
Green Drink or Chlorophyll, Bee Pollen, Brewers Yeast, Mineral
Water.
   No sugar, refined foods.

# IMPETIGO

Impetigo is a fungal infection.
—Apply Black Walnut tincture to sores. May use internally.
—Apply Garlic oil to affected area, can take internally also.
—Salt baths can help dry up sores. 1 cup salt per tub of water.
—Take Infection Fighting Combination #2 orally.

# INFERTILITY—IMPOTENCY
(See Vitamin E, Selenium and Zinc sections)

(For men—see Prostate sections, For women— see also Infertility
section in For Women Only.)

**Herbal Combinations:**

Infection Fighting Combination #2        Prostate Combinations
Infertility—Impotency Combination

**Single Herbs:**

| | | |
|---|---|---|
| Chickweed | **Ginseng** | **Sage** |
| Cornsilk | **Goldenseal** | **Sarsaparilla** |
| Damiana | Licorice | **Taheebo** |

**Vitamins & Minerals:** Natural Multiple Vit. & Min. Supplement
   **Vitamin E with Selenium, Zinc,** Mega A, C. All minerals.
**Diet:** Real Food Diet, Juice Fasts, Mild Food Diet, Green Drink or
chlorophyll, Bee Pollen, Eat Selenium-rich and Zinc-rich foods. See
minerals.
   —Many times this problem can be corrected just by improving the
diet to a wholesome one. Junk Food Diets have been a contributing
factor to many an impotency problem.

# INSOMNIA—SLEEPLESSNESS

**Herbal Combinations:**

Nerve and Relaxing Combinations        Sleepy Tea Combinations

**Single Herbs:**

Camomile            **Comfrey tea**           Lobelia
**Cascara Sagrada**     **Hops tea**

**Vitamins & Minerals:** Natural Multiple Vit. & Min. Supplement
    B Vitamins, take in the day time. Calcium, take before bedtime.
**Diet:** Real Food Diet, No junk food, etc. (See Hyperactivity this
chapter.)
**Other:** Exercise and Chiropractic care both help.
    —Do not exercise just before going to bed. Go to bed when sleepy,
but get up the usual time in the morning no matter how much sleep.
Body will usually regulate itself.

# KIDNEY/BLADDER

**Herbal Combinations:**

Kidney/Bladder Combs.      Infection Fighting Comb. plus Garlic

**Single Herbs:**

| | | |
|---|---|---|
| Alfalfa | **Cornsilk** | Peach Bark |
| Aloe Vera | **Dandelion** | Poke Root |
| Barberry | **Echinacea** | **Red Raspberry** |
| Black Cohosh | Fennel | **Safflower** |
| Blessed Thistle | **Goldenseal** | Sage |
| Blue Cohosh | Horsetail | Slippery Elm |
| Burdock | Juniper Berries | **Taheebo** |
| **Catnip** | **Kelp** | **Uva Ursi** |
| Cayenne | Licorice Root | White Oak Bark |
| Camomile | **Marshmallow** | **Yarrow** |
| Chaparral | **Parsley** | Yellow Dock |
| **Comfrey** | | |

**Vitamins & Minerals:** Natural Multiple Vit. & Min. Supplement
    B Complex, Choline, Mega A, C, E. Treat as cold.

**Diet:** Real Food Diet, Juice Fast, Mild Food Diet, Chlorophyll or Green Drink, Aloe Vera Juice, **Cranberry juice, or cranberry apple juice, Lemon juice,** Watermelon juice. Apple Cider Vinegar 2 Tb. to 1 glass water with meals.

# KIDNEY STONES

—Drink juice of ½ fresh lemon in 8 ounce glass of water every ½ hour or hour until pain subsides. Can alternate lemon juice and apple juice.
   —Take kidney combination. (See also Kidneys this chapter)
   —Take Pain Combination.
   —1000 mg. Vitamin C every hour.
   —Take warm catnip enema when pain subsides.
   —It takes 5 to 14 hours to dissolve stones.
Note: As a preventative drink juice of ½ lemon in glass of warm water first thing each morning, drink cranberry juice or cranberry apple juice each day.

# LARYNGITIS—SEE HOARSENESS

# LEUCORRHEA—See For Women Only

# LIVER—See also Hepatitis

**Herbal Combinations:**

Liver/Gall Combinations

**Single Herbs:**

| | | |
|---|---|---|
| **Aloe Vera Juice** | Cayenne | Parsley |
| Barberry | | Redmond Clay |
| Bayberry | **Dandelion** | Sage Taheebo |
| Black Cohosh | Fennel | Uva Ursi |
| Blessed Thistle | Garlic | White Oak Bark |
| Buckthorn | Goldenseal | Wood Betony |
| Burdock | Horsetail | **Yarrow** |
| **Cascara Sagrada** | Lobelia | **Yellow Dock** |

**Vitamins & Minerals:** Natural Multiple Vit. & Min. Supplement B Complex, Choline, Mega A, C, E. Treat as cold.

**Diet:** Real Food Diet, Mild Food Diet, Juice Fast, Chlorophyll or Green Drink—include Dandelion in Green Drink. **Lemon or Apple Juice Fast**, Beet Juice, Bee Pollen.

## LOW BLOOD PRESSURE—See Blood Pressure

## LYMPHATIC SYSTEM

**Herbal Combinations:**

Infection Fighting Comb. #2          Blood Purifying Combinations

**Single Herbs:**

| | | |
|---|---|---|
| **Burdock** | **Goldenseal** | **Poke Root** |
| **Echinacea** | **Myrrh** | **Yarrow** |
| | | **Yellow Dock** |

**Vitamins & Minerals:** Natural Multiple Vit. & Min. Supplement
   B Complex, Pantothenic Acid, Mega A, C, E. Treat as cold.
**Diet:** Real Food Diet, Juice Fast, Mild Food Diet, Chlorophyll or Green Drink.
**Other:** Catnip/Garlic Enema
**Exercise:** important, jogging or others. **Mini-Trampoline.**

## MEASLES—See Childhood Diseases, Baby Chapter

## MENOPAUSE—See For Women Only

## MONONUCLEOSIS

Good nutrition to help build the body needs to be first priority in mononucleosis. Follow instructions in diet section below.

**Herbal Combinations:**

Infection Fighting Combinations

**Single Herbs:**

| | | |
|---|---|---|
| Burdock | Cayenne | Dandelion |

| | | |
|---|---|---|
| **Echinacea** | Goldenseal | **Poke Root** |
| **Garlic** | Myrrh | Yellow Dock |
| | | **Yarrow** |

**Vitamins & Minerals:** Natural Multiple Vit. & Min. Supplement B Complex, Choline, Mega A, C, E. Treat as cold. Large doses of Vitamin C have been successfully used to help this problem. Remember to give B Complex and Calcium if large doses of C are used.
**Diet:** Real Food Diet, Juice Fast, Mild Food Diet, Chlorophyll or Green Drink, Fresh juices, sprouts, soups, (acute illness diet this chapter) Bee Pollen.

## MOTION SICKNESS

— 2 to 3 capsules Ginger or Ginger tea taken several hours before an air trip or drive in cars has helped. Repeat as needed.
— Flu Combination #1, which is largely Ginger, has also been effective when taken the same as above.
— Taking B vitamins on a regular basic help prevent motion sickness.
— Chinese Herbal Oils. Dip a toothpick in oil and put toothpick in mouth or put a few drops oil in small glass water and drink.

## MUMPS—See Childhood Diseases, Baby Chapter

## MUCUS

Note: If there is mucus in sinus, head, throat or lung area, the body is probably overloaded with it throughout the whole digestive system.
— Treat this as a cold, with particular emphasis where the mucus is. For instance in the head and sinus, treat as a cold and as allergies or sinus. If in the lungs, treat as a cold or as Bronchitis, etc.
— Clean colon—Catnip/Garlic enema. Juice Fasts.

## MULTIPLE SCLEROSIS

**Herbal Combinations:**

Nerve and Relaxing Combinations

**Single Herbs:**

Lobelia

**Vitamins & Minerals:** Natural Multiple Vit. & Min. Supplement B Complex, Pantothenic Acid, Mega A, C, E. Lecithin, **Calcium, and all minerals.**

**Diet:** Real Food Diet, Juice Fast, Mild Food Diet, Chlorophyll or Green Drink, emphasis on sprouts, raw foods, homemade cottage cheese, whey, raw honey for sweetener.

No sugar, coffee, chocolate, or refined foods.

**Other:** Keep colon clean.

— Exercise, swimming

— Massage

## MUSCLE SPASM

— Rub externally with Lobelia extract.

— Vinegar/salt baths.

— Calcium, Magnesium, Manganese. B Vitamins.

— Nerve and Relaxing Combinations.

## NAILS—RIDGED, BRITTLE ETC.

**Herbal Combinations:**

Hair, Skin and Nails Combinations          Calcium Combinations

**Single Herbs:**

| | | |
|---|---|---|
| **Alfalfa** | **Kelp** | Parsley |
| **Dandelion** | **Horsetail** | **Yellow Dock** |

**Vitamins & Minerals:** Natural Multiple Vit. & Min. Supplements **Zinc, and trace minerals.**

**Diet:** Real Food Diet, Mineral water.

## NEPHRITIS—See also Kidneys

— 1 cup Marshmallow/Red Raspberry tea or Cornsilk tea every 3 or 4 hours.

— Drinking as much raw goat milk (raw cow's milk may be substituted but is not as good) a day as one can (2 or 4 qts) will often clear up kidney problems. This can be done with the Mild Food Diet or as a Milk Fast.

— Kidney Combinations, Infection Fighting Combinations
— Lobelia, Golden Seal. **Treat as cold**
— Cleanse colon
— Catnip/Garlic enemas.

## NOSE BLEEDS

— Take 2 cayenne capsules by mouth.
— Re-occurring nose bleeds are often caused by a B Vitamin deficiency.

## NURSING—See Pregnancy Chapter

## OBESITY—WEIGHT LOSS

**Herbal Combinations:**
Weight Loss Combination plus Chickweed
Lower Bowel Combination to prevent constipation
Kidney/Bladder Combinations for water retention
Calcium Combinations

**Single Herbs:**

| | | |
|---|---|---|
| **Cascara Sagrada** | Fennel | Safflower |
| **Chickweed** | **Kelp** | Yarrow |
| Dandelion | Papaya | |
| Echinacea | Parsley | |

**Vitamins & Minerals:** Natural Multiple Vit. & Min. Supplement B Complex, C, E, Lecithin, Calcium, Magnesium.
**Diet:** Real Food Diet, Juice Fast, Mild Food Diet, Chlorophyll or Green Drink. — Emphasis on whole, unprocessed foods tend to tell the brain that you are not hungry and can lower the weight regulating mechanism in the brain. Refined foods and junk food, on the other hand, tells the brain you need more nourishment so the brain sends hunger signals to you.
**Exercise:** Helps to keep metabolism of the thyroid up.

# OBSTRUCTED BOWELS—See also Constipation

— Turkey Rhubarb tea has been effective in helping blockages; drink as much tea as possible until blockage is gone. May cause profuse diarrhea. Can also use Turkey Rhubarb enemas. If bowels are very obstructed may also need massage therapy and/or colonics. This is a purgative, do not use if pregnant.

# OSTEOPOROSIS (Severe, porosity of bones)

**Herbal Combinations:**
Calcium Combinations                Hair, Skin and Nails Combinations

**Single Herbs:**

Alfalfa              **Dandelion**              **Kelp**
**Comfrey**

**Vitamins & Minerals:** Natural Multilple Vit. & Min. Supplement
   **Calcium,** Phosphorus, Magnesium, Mega A, **C, D,** E, **B Vitamins.**
Mineral Water, (See Calcium section.)
**Diet:** Real Food Diet, Mild Food Diet, Chlorophyll or Green Drink, salads, soups, homemade cottage cheese, Digestive Enzymes. **Emphasis on raw juices, especially carrot.**

No sugar or refined foods; avoid meat, especially beef.

# OVARIES—See For Women Only

# PARASITES—WORMS

— Apple Juice Fast for 3 days. Take Garlic after juice fast.

**Herbal Combinations:**
General Cleanser and Parasite Combination
Parasite Combination
Lower Bowel Combination

**Single Herbs:**

| | | |
|---|---|---|
| **Aloe Vera juice** | **Cascara Sagrada** | Horsetail |
| **Black Walnut** | Catnip | Juniper Berries |
| Blessed Thistle | Chamomile | Kelp |
| Buckthorn | **Garlic** | Lobelia |

| Papaya | Sage | White Oak Bark |
| Peach Bark | Slippery Elm | White Willow |
| Red Raspberry | Thyme | Wood Betony |
| Redmond Clay | Valerian Root | |

**Vitamins & Minerals:** Natural Multiple Vit. & Min. Supplement
Take after Juice fast not during it.
**Other:** Garlic Enema.

— Drinking Aloe Vera juice has helped expel pin worms.

# PARKINSON'S DISEASE

Diet and herbs have been known to help alleviate symptoms, but as of yet no cure has been found.

**Herbal Combinations:**
Energy and Memory Combinations Nerve and Relaxing Combinations

**Single Herbs:**

Cayenne                Ginseng

**Vitamins & Minerals:** Natural Multiple Vit. & Min. Supplement
**B Complex, B6,** Mega C, E, Lecithin, Calcium, Magnesium, Zinc, Lithium.
**Diet:** Real Food Diet, Short Juice Fasts, 5 or 6 days, Mild Food Diet, Chlorophyll or Green Drink, Bee Pollen, Aloe Vera juice, Brewer's Yeast, raw fruits juices, raw goats milk, sprouts.

# PITUITARY

**Herbal Combinations:**
Blood Builder Combinations

**Single Herbs**

| **Alfalfa** | **Gotu Kola** | **Parsley** |
| **Ginseng** | **Kelp** | Yellow Dock |

**Vitamins & Minerals:** Natural Multiple Vit. & Min. Supplements
Trace Minerals.

**Diet:** Real Food Diet, Chlorophyll or Green Drink, and other foods high in minerals such as sprouts, juices, etc.

# PLEURISY

Pleurisy pack: 3 heaping Tb. Slippery Elm, 1 Tb. Lobelia, ½ tsp. Cayenne. Mix with distilled or plain water. Can be left on chest all night. Sometimes packs for the chest need to be put on the back as well as the front.

# PNEUMONIA—See Bronchitis

# POISON IVY OR OAK

— Cleanse system, treat as for cold, Juice Fast.
— Aloe Vera ointment, gel or juice topically. Can drink also.
— Black Walnut tincture or Chinese Herbal oils topically.
— For more on itching see Bee Stings.

**Herbal Combinations:**
Blood Purifier Combination #1

**Single Herbs:**

| | | |
|---|---|---|
| **Aloe Vera Juice** | Burdock | Slippery Elm |
| **Black Walnut** | Lobelia | Yellow Dock |

# PROSTATE—See also INFERTILITY

**Herbal Combinations:**
Prostate Combinations      Infection Fighting Combinations
(See also Prostate Combination)

**Single Herbs:**

| | | |
|---|---|---|
| Damiana | **Goldenseal** | **Parsley** |
| **Echinacea** | Kelp | Saw Palmetto |
| Ginseng | Juniper Berries | |

**Vitamins & Minerals:** Natural Multiple Vit. & Min. Supplement
   B Complex, Mega A, C, E, Vitamin F, Lecithin, Potassium, Man-

ganese, Zinc, Selenium. Zinc and Selenium are very important in
helping to prevent and alleviate prostate problems. Just increasing
zinc has helped some men to stop having problems with needing to
get up at night and having little or no stream.(See also Vitamin E,
Selenium, and Zinc in Vitamin an Mineral Chapter.)
**Diet:** Real Food Diet, Juice Fast, Bee Pollen, Pumpkin Seeds,
Chlorophyll or green drink, Brewer's Yeast.
**Other:** Garlic enemas
**Exercise:** Walking, Jogging.

# PSORIASIS

Chronic, non-contagious skin disease. Has white, scaly patches
and inflamation.

**Herbal Combinations:**
Blood Purifier Combinations

**Single Herbs:**

| | | |
|---|---|---|
| **Aloe Vera, external** | Comfrey | Sarsaparilla |
| **Burdock** | **Dandelion** | Slippery Elm |
| Chaparral | Kelp | Taheebo |
| Chickweed | Red Clover | **Yellow Dock** |

**Vitamins & Minerals:** Natural Multiple Vit. & Min. Supplement
    **A**, C, **D**, E, B Complex, **Lecithin,** Calcium, Potassium, **Zinc. Many
people who have psoriasis have problems assimilating vitamins,
expecially A. Find the easiest vitamins to assimilate available.**
**Diet:** Real Food Diet, Juice Fast, Mild Food diet, Juice fast, Mild
Food Diet, Chlorophyll or Green Drink. Emphasis on raw foods. Use
digestive enzymes with meals. Brewer's Yeast, Bee Pollen, Wheat
Grass, Barley Green.
    No refined foods or sugar.

# PYORRHEA

Gum inflammation developing into possible tooth loss, because of
loose teeth.

**Herbal Combinations:**
Rinse mouth with Poultice Combination. (See also Cankers)

**Single Herbs**

| | | |
|---|---|---|
| **Aloe Vera juice** | Cayenne | **Goldenseal** |
| Barberry | Chlorophyll | Lobelia |
| **Bayberry** | Comfrey | Myrrh |

**Vitamins & Minerals:** Natural Multiple Vit. & Min. Supplements Mega A, **C,** E. Large doses of Vitamin C have been effectively used, even in cases where teeth were almost going to be lost. Can also rinse mouth with Mineral water.

**Diet:** Real Food Diet, Mild Food Diet, Chlorophyll or Green Drink.

# RHEUMATISM—See Arthritis

# RINGWORM

— Black Walnut tincture, Aloe Vera juice or gel, comfrey tincture, Oil of Garlic, or Apple cider vinegar can all be used topically. Can be taken internally also.

— Poultices of Lobelia or Goldenseal are effective. These herbs can also be taken internally.

— Taheebo is used internally and externally.

# SCARLET FEVER—Treat as for acute illness

# SCARLETINA—Treat as acute illness—See Baby section

# SCARS

— **Vitamin E** and **Aloe Vera**—internally and externally. Castor Oil and Olive Oil—externally. Apply any of these four externally, liberally. (See also Vitamin E)

— Massaging scar tissue while rubbing in one of the above has been known to help heal the tissue, lessen the scarring, and give more movement, even in old scar tissue.

— Taking Poultice Combination by mouth after an injury has helped better healing and less scarring.

— Wheat Grass, Barley Grass for scars in lungs.

# SENILITY

Seniliy is often caused by vitamin and mineral deficiencies rather than just "old age". We suggest you reread the Vitamin and Mineral Chapter paying close attention to the deficiency sections.

**Herbal Combinations:**
Energy and Memory Combinations

**Single Herbs:**

| | | |
|---|---|---|
| Cayenne | Ginseng | Gotu Kola, |
| Dandelion | | concentrated |

**Vitamins & Minerals:** Natural Multiple Vit. & Min. Supplements
All Vitamins and minerals important especially **B vitamins,** Inositol, Choline (Lecithin).
**Diet:** Real Food Diet, Mild Food Diet, Chlorophyll or Green Drink, Raw juices, Bee Pollen.
No refined foods, sugar or salt.
**Other:** Positive Thinking and keeping the mind active and alert is essential to the prevention of senility.

# SHINGLES

— Nerve and Relaxing Combinations
— B Vitamins, Vitamin A, Minerals especially Calcium and Zinc.
— Apple cider vinegar dabbed on sore areas has been used to relieve pain for 1 to 2 hours.
— Chinese Herbal oils.
— See also itching.
— See also itching under Mosquito and Spider Bites, p. 195.

# SHOCK

— **Cayenne**-1 to 3 tsp stirred in warm water or 2 to 4 capsules. Take by mouth. Cayenne tincture is excellent to keep on hand or in the car in case of emergencies. It can be dribbled in the mouth even if the person is not able to sit to swallow. ½ tsp Tincture can also be used in warm water.
for child: 1 or 2 capsules, 1 tsp stirred in warm water, or ¼ tsp tincture.

for baby: use ⅛ tincture, ¼ tsp powdered, or 1 capsule stirred in warm water.

## SINUSES—Treat as cold

**Sinus Washes:**

1. Boil 1 pint water, cool, add 1 tsp salt, 1 tsp soda, 1 Tb. Witch Hazel. Snuff up one nostril at a time an spit out. This loosens the hard mucous material in sinus and cleans it out when nothing else will. Can be done several times a day.

2. Goldenseal tea snuffed up nostrils or used as nosedrops. This is also good for babies and children.

3. Place 1 tsp. Chia seeds on tongue and swallow with glass of water.

**Other:** — 1000 mg. of C an hour helps to loosen mucus in sinus.

— 50,000 to 100,000 IU of Vitamin A day acts as a natural antihistamine.

— Pantothenic Acid can help rid the problem and prevent it from happening again.

— Chinese Oils.

## SMOKING

**Herbal Combinations:**

Blood Builder Combinations        Lung Combinations

Nerve and Relaxing Combinations

**Single Herbs:**

| | | |
|---|---|---|
| **Dandelion** | Kelp | **Scullcap** |
| **Echinacea** | **Licorice** | **Valerian Root** |
| Goldenseal | Lobelia | |
| **Hops** | Peppermint | |

**Vitamins & Minerals:** Natural Multiple Vit. & Min. Supplement **B Complex,** Mega **A, C,** E. **All minerals.**

**Diet:** Real Food Diet, Juice Fast, Mild Food Diet, Chlorophyll or Green Drink. Juice fasts help to break the habit of any drugs that are addictive.

## SPRAINS, SWELLINGS, PULLED TENDONS

— Ice packs, onion poultices, comfrey poultices, Poultice Combination poultices, plantain poultices, Hot fomentations of Burdock. See also Bruises.

— Chinese Herbal Oils.

## STOMACH ACHE

Drink 1 or 2 ounces of Aloe Vera juice.

— 15-25 drops (adults) of Catnip/Fennel tincture in ¼ cup warm water. (2-3 drops newborns, 3-6 drops up to 3 or 6 months. Increase drops as child grows in size or need to 12 to 15 drops for older child.) This may be repeated as necessary but it is usually best to wait 10 to 20 minutes to give it time to work. If the pain is severe repeat dose sooner. Often after giving Catnip/Fennel the person or baby will start to burp until much gas is relieved. After using this a few times you will become comfortable with how much and how often is effective for your family.

— Peppermint tea or oil of peppermint.

— 1 to 3 drops Chinese Herbal Oils in 2 ounces water. Children 1 to 2 drops. These can also be rubbed on the stomach.

## TETANUS—Treat as for acute illness

**Herbal Combinations:**
Nerve Combination
Infection Fighting Combinations

**Single Herbs:** All anti-spasmodic herbs.

| | | |
|---|---|---|
| Black Cohosh | Hops | Scullcap |
| Catnip | **Lobelia** | Valerian Root, |
| Cayenne | Mistletoe |    extract |
| Fennel | Passion Flower | Wood Betony |

**Vitamins & Minerals:** Natural Multiple Vit. & Min. Supplement B Complex, Mega A, C, E.

**Diet:** Real Food Diet, Juice Fast, mostly vegetables and green drink.

## THRUSH—See Yeast Infection, Baby Chapter

# TONSILLITIS OR SORE THROAT—Treat as for Cold

— Take bottle of glycerine, add enough iodine to make it a dark amber color. Use to swab tonsils 1 to 3 times a day. This is also good for strep throat. The glycerine holds the iodine to the throat and the iodine kills the germs.

— Open Infection Fighting Combination #2, put in juice or water and drink. Will fight infection and help take pain out of throat. Can also be taken in capsules, if bathing the throat isn't necessary.

— dissolve oil of garlic pearl in mouth or use garlic extract.

— Hold sliced garlic bud in mouth between teeth and cheek for 2 to 8 hours and let juice go down throat. This fights infection and takes pain out of throat very quickly. The garlic will make the mouth a little sore where it has been held, but this soreness will go away within 24 hours or so.

— Onion packs around neck. Leave on overnight. See Herbal Recipes.

— Swallow small amounts of aloe vera juice, or pineapple juice.

— 1000 mg. Vitamin C every hour.

— White Willow use for aspirin.

— ¼ tsp. Cayenne stirred in water. Drink every 2 or 3 hours. (or can take 1 to 2 capsules)

— 1 tsp. chlorophyll in ½ C. water, gargle.

**Note:** Infection Fighting Combinations by mouth, Treat as cold.

# THYROID

**Herbal Combinations:**
Thyroid Combinations                    Nerve and Relaxing Combinations

**Single Herbs:**

**Kelp**

**Vitamins & Minerals:** Natural Multiple Vit. & Min. Supplement B Complex, Mega A, C, E. **Iodine.**

**Diet:** Real Food Diet, Mild Food Diet, Chlorophyll or Green Drink.

# TOOTHACHE

— Rub 1 or 2 drops of Chinese Herbal Oil topically on area.
— 2 or 3 drops of lobelia.

# TOOTH EXTRACTION OR ORAL SURGERY

Rinse mouth with warm tea made of equals parts of Goldenseal and White Oak Bark as needed for pain, swelling, or bleeding.

# ULCERS—COLITIS—DIVERTICULITIS

**Herbal Combinations:**
Ulcer Combination          Colitis Combination plus Slippery Elm

**Single Herbs:**

| | | |
|---|---|---|
| **Aloe Vera juice** | Garlic | **Peppermint Tea** |
| Bayberry | Ginger | Psyllium |
| Black Walnut | **Goldenseal** | **Slippery Elm** |
| Camomile | Kelp | Taheebo |
| Comfrey | Myrrh | |

**Vitamins & Minerals:** Natural Multiple Vit. & Min. Supplement B Complex, Mega A, C, E, Vitamin K and U. All Minerals.
**Diet:** Real Food Diet, Mild Food Diet, Chlorophyll or Green Diet, Aloe Vera juice, Mineral water, Acidolphilus, Digestive Enzymes.
**Cabbage and cabbage juice** (see Vitamin U)
**Other:** Cleanse colon, reduce stress, use postive thinking.
**Colitis helps:** See enemas for Slippery Elm enemas and Mineral Water enemas. Also colonics are good. Some believe Colitis is a deficiency disease of Vitamin K. (See Vitamin K.)
**Ulcer helps:**
— Raw Cabbage Juice, See Vitamin U.
— Take 2 capsules Ulcer Combination plus 2 capsules Slippery Elm ½ hour before meals. Can be taken with mineral water or aloe vera juice.
— Drink 1 ounce mineral water or 1 to 2 ounces aloe vera juice ½ hour before meal. These drinks can be alternated.
— 2 capsules Poultice Combination before meals. This combination contains Aloe Vera and Slippery Elm among others excellent healing herbs.

# VARICOSE VEINS

**Herbal Combinations:**
Liver/Gall Combination              Goldenseal/White Oak Bark

**Single Herbs:**

| | | |
|---|---|---|
| Cayenne | **Goldenseal** | Lobelia |
| Comfrey | Kelp | **White Oak Bark** |

— Eight capsules a day of White Oak Bark has helped control and alleviate symptoms of varicose veins.

**Vitamins & Minerals:** Natural Multiple Vit. & Min. Supplements
    B Complex, Rutin, Mega A, C, E.
**Diet:** Real Food Diet, Mild Food Diet, Chlorophyll or Green Drink
**Other:**
    — Goldenseal/White Oak Bark fomentations are one of the better remedies.
    — Vinegar fomentations
    — Marigold tea fomentations. Make from petals of marigolds
    — Comfrey poultices.

(See case history—White Oak Bark)

# VOMITING-See Flu-Influenza

# WARTS

— Put milk from milkweed plant on wart. Repeat each day until wart goes away. Depending on the size of the wart it can take a few days or a few weeks.
    — **Seed Wart.** Fresh Aloe Vera. Peel leaf and leave pulp. Put the pulp on wart, wrap with cloth or use band aid to hold. Leave overnight. One night may be enough or it may need to be repeated for several weeks, depending again on size and stubbornness of the wart.
    — Put castor oil on first-then apply slice of raw garlic to area. Leave overnight. usually takes about 3 weeks.
    — Vitamin A and E on wart and take internally with a good multiple. Note: People who get warts often are usually deficient in Vitamin A.

# WOUNDS, CUTS, ABRASIONS

— Apply cayenne to stop bleeding or take cayenne by mouth. See bleeding.

— Poultice Combination, can be used for minor or more severe cuts that don't require stitches. Has even been used in some cases instead of stitches when medical help was not available. I have also mixed this powder into Comfrey salve or other creams and used it on a band aid instead of making a poultice. See also Bruises.

— Comfrey salves are wonderful to stop pain, and fight infection for minor cuts and abrasions. I like the ones best that also have Chickweed and other healing herbs in with it.

# YEAST INFECTION-See For Women Only

# YELLOW JAUNDICE (Non-Infectious)

**Herbal Combinations:**

Liver/Gall Combinations

**Single Herbs:**

| | | |
|---|---|---|
| Barberry | **Dandelion** | Slippery Elm |
| Bayberry | Fennel | Wood Betony |
| **Cascara Sagrada** | Horsetail | **Yarrow** |
| **Cayenne** | Parsley | **Yellow Dock** |
| Chamomile | Peach Bark | |

**Vitamins & Minerals:** Natural Multiple Vit. & Min. Supplement B Complex, Mega A, C, E. Treat as cold. For more about Vitamin E and Jaundice see Baby Chapter under Jaundice.
**Diet:** Real Food Diet, Juice Fast, Mild Food Diet, Chlorophyll or Green drink, Carrot and Beet Juice.
**Other:** Enemas- Catnip/Garlic, and Cayenne.
**For Jaundice in a baby—See Baby Chapter**

# CHAPTER 10

# *Herbal Preparations and Herbal Recipes*

## HERBAL PREPARATIONS

Herbs can be used as teas, extracts, poultices, etc., as well as in the newer forms such as capsules and concentrated capsules.

Herbs used in infusions or teas are in solution and contain only the water soluble parts that can be extracted by pouring boiling water over the dried, powdered, or fresh herb.

**The advantages of teas are:**

1. They are easily assimilated, easier for a weak body to accept.
2. The hot water helps release the power of the herb.
3. Liquid is already in the tea.

Capsuled herbs are capsuled in gelatin capsules, which dissolve very quickly. They are concentrated and contain both water soluble and oil soluble parts of the herb since the whole herb is ground and capsuled. Note: Capsules should be taken with a glass of water.

**The advantages of capsuled herbs are:**

1. Contains both oil soluble and water soluble parts of the herb.
2. More convenient form to take and carry, so more people are consistent in taking what they need.
3. Many of the most medicinal herbs are the most bitter. Taking them in capsule form makes them more convenient and more palatable.

## How to Prepare or Buy Them

**Infusion—**      Tea made from leaves, stems, blossoms, or powdered herb. Pour 1 cup boiling water over 1 Tb. of *fresh* herb; 1 tsp. *dried* herb; 1 tsp. *powdered* herb **or** open 4 capsules. Cover, and let steep 10 to 20 minutes. Never boil.

**Decoction—**      Tea made from bark and roots. Put 2 Tb. cut pieces per 1 cup cold water. Bring to a slight, gentle boil and gently simmer for 20 to 30 minutes. Strain. Reuse the same herbs with another cup cold water and repeat the above process. Strain. Mix both batches together.

**Compress or Fomentation—**      Dip clean cloth into warm infusion or decoction. Wring out and apply to affected areas. Used for swellings, pain, colds, flu, inflammations, hemorrhoids, varicose veins, etc. Better used when warm and allowed to cool on the body. Reapply as needed.

**Extracts or Tinctures—**      Herbs aged in alcohol or apple cider vinegar. Put 4 oz. powdered herb or 8 ozs. dried herb to 1 pint apple cider vinegar or alcohol. (Everclear brand 190 proof is a good one.) Shake bottle 2 times daily and allow it to age from 12-14 days. Powdered herbs only take 4 or 5 days. Aging herbs in alcohol extracts more of the properties than does vinegar. It also mixes easier when putting tinctures or extracts in juices. Putting the dosage of alcohol tincture in about ¼ cup very warm water will dissipate the alcohol. These herbal preparations are easily assimilated and much more concentrated than the herb alone.

**Oils of Herbs**      Herbs extracted in oil. Pound dried or fresh herb. Add 1 pint olive oil to 2 oz. of herb and let it sit in a warm place for 4 days or put mixture in a double boiler and gently heat oil for 1 or 2 hours. Press oil from herb. Some vitamin E may be added to help preserve it. Store in bottle in refrigerator.

**Ointment or Salves**

Warm a natural vaseline product or lanolin. Stir in enough powdered herbs to bring mixture to a dark color. Pour in containers when cool but still pliable and let it set.

**Bolus—**

An internal poultice to be used as a suppository in vaginal or rectal area. For instructions on how to make see Other Remedies in For Women Only section.

**Capsules—**

Herbs for different ailments are available in capsules. As long as the capsuled herbs are kept dry they store indefinitely.

**Concentrated Herbs in Capsules—**

These are herbal extracts that have been freeze-dried, removing the moisture content, but leaving the healing elements. The result is a highly concentrated capsuled form. **One capsule of the concentrated herb equals four of the regular herb.**

**Poultice**

Herbs chopped, blended, grated, or powdered and applied to external swellings, wounds, etc. If using powdered herb mix first with mineral water and then olive oil or castor oil and apply directly to wound. If using fresh herb blend in blender with small amount of mineral water and put prepared herb in soft, clean cloth. Apply cloth or herbs next to skin—cover outer part of poultice with plastic wrap to keep from soiling clothes or bedding. Used for swellings, inflammations, wounds, stings, bites, chest colds, and in some cases certain herbs will actually pull foreign matter from wounds, scrapes, etc.

# HERBAL RECIPES

## BATHS

One of the body's most important eliminating organs is the skin. Baths help bring out toxins through the pores, promote perspiration, help to bring down fevers, and are relaxing and soothing for sore muscles, bruises, etc. Stay in water 20 to 30 minutes.
— Ginger Bath. 3 to 4 Tb. to tepid bath water.
— Vinegar/Salt. 1 cup Vinegar, ½ cup salt to tepid bath water.
— Salt Bath. 1 cup salt in bath tub of water.
— Chickweed, Comfrey Baths for sores and rashes. 2 qts. tea per tub of water.

## CIDER DRINK (SWEET AND SOUR DRINK)

1-2 tsp. of apple cider vinegar and 1-2 tsp. honey in glass of water (warm or cool). Drink 2 or 3 times daily for healthful benefits. A pleasant tasting drink, can be used as a beverage with a meal or 20-30 minutes before a meal, for digestion problems.

## COUGH SYRUPS

### Cayenne and Ginger Cough Syrup

¼ tsp Cayenne, ¼ tsp Ginger, 1 Tb. honey, 1 Tb. vinegar. Mix with 2 Tb. hot water. Take as needed.

### Lemon/Honey Syrup

Use fresh lemon juice, honey and water in proportions that taste good to you. Warm in pan until honey is dissolved. Delicious drunk warm or cold. Good for singers to use to help throats when fighting sore throats.

### Grandmother's Cough Syrup

¼ cup honey, juice of 1 lemon, ½ tsp Ginger, alum size of pea. Add a little water if needed. Heat to together and serve warm.

**Mom's Cough Syrup**

Slice 2 large onions, drizzle ½ lemon juice and 1 Tb. honey over the onion. Turn to lowest heat and pour off juice as it comes out. Makes about 1 cup cough syrup. This usually takes about 45 minutes to an hour to get all the juice out.

## MUSTARD PLASTERS

1. **For children and babies** can be left on over night without burning. However any age can use it. 1 Tb. Ginger, 1 Tb. dry mustard, 1 Tb. turpentine, 1 Tb. salt, 3 Tb. lard or shortening. Mix together. Spread in soft cloth and apply to chest.
2. 1 Tb. dry mustard, 4 Tb. flour, 1 egg. Mix with water and **leave until skin is pink.**
3. 10 level Tb. flour, 1 level Tb. dry mustard. Mix with water. Leave on for about **15 minutes** or **until skin is pink.**
*Note:* For 2 and 3 put vaseline on chest before applying pack.

## PACKS

**Onion pack:** Used for infection, chest, soreness, bruises, swelling, etc.

**Potato pack:** Used for liver, kidneys, tumors, etc.
Grate onion or potatoe lay in cloth, apply to affected area.

**Clay pack:** Used for kidneys, burns, tumors, infection, pain, skin, etc.
Mix clay with mineral water until pasty and apply.

## POULTICES

Poultice Combination can be used or healing herbs of your choosing. It is a good idea to mix Slippery Elm in a poultice if you make your own, because it helps hold the other herbs together. For instructions on how to make see Herbal Preparations.

# SALVES

**Comfrey Salve:** can be purchased. Salves with Comfrey and Chickweed (and other healing herbs) are wonderful because of the contact healing properties of those herbs.

**Poultice Combination Salve:** mix poultice combination in with another salve, comfrey, or an A and E cream, or with natural vaseline.

**Goldenseal/Myrrh Salve:** Mix Goldenseal and Myrrh in equal parts in a natural vaseline until it becomes a dark color.

# CHAPTER 11

# Survival, Year's Supply

## SURVIVAL OR YEAR'S SUPPLY

**Herbs** are essential to a year's supply. Herbs store indefinitely as long as they are kept in a cool, dry place. They are good to have on hand for camping, etc. Study and learn all you can since you need to know how to use them.

**Vitamins and Minerals** are essential to store. Most everything we store is canned. The vitamin content of canned foods is low and contains no vitamin C which humans need daily. Vitamins are also needed for stress. If they are going to be used during illness they are needed in mega-doses.

**Seeds** are essential. They can be sprouted so one can have fresh foods within 3 days. (alfalfa, lentils, pinto beans, radishes, etc.)

## HERBAL SURVIVAL LIST

1. Cayenne-shock, bleeding etc.
2. Peppermint and Catnip leaves - for tea/enemas, fever etc.
3. Garlic capsules - fights infection enemas, etc.
4. Aloe Vera juice and gel - stomach aches, burns, etc.
5. Slippery Elm-diarrhea
6. Infection fighting herbs and combinations, (natural antibiotics)
7. Poultice combinations - for cuts, wounds, burns, etc.
8. Allergy herbs or combinations
9. Lobelia tincture - relaxing, spasms, etc.
10. Ginger - for baths, remedies.

11. Multiple vitamin, infection fighting vitamins C, A, E, Pantothenic acid - for mega-therapy.
12. Comfrey tincture, capsules, or leaves.
13. Mineral water - antiseptic, sores in mouth, mix with poultice, remedies, etc.
14. Castor oil, olive oil - remedies.
15. Eucalyptus oil - for steaming.
16. Apple cider vinegar - baths, remedies
17. Salt, shortening, turpentine - for remedies
18. Dry mustard - mustard plasters
19. Untreated seeds for sprouting or planting - (wheat, alfalfa, lentil, radish, chives, parsley, watercress, spinach, cabbage, carrots, spinach, cucumbers, pinto beans, white beans)
20. Onions - for packs and remedies.
21. Spirulina - good source of protein, vitamins, minerals.
22. Apple cider vinegar - digestion, baths, etc.
23. Water purification
    a. Water tablets
    b. Tincture of iodine - Boil water. 12 drops to 1 gal clear water, or 24 drops for cloudy water.
24. Water conditioner (don't confuse this with water softeners that use salt.)
25. Cloths and cotton for poultices, bandages, etc.
26. Thermometer and alcohol
27. Enema bags
28. Your own personal needs or favorites.

CHAPTER **12**

# *Exercise*

## EXERCISE

Paavo Airola stated that if he had to choose between someone who ate well and didn't exercise or someone who didn't eat well but exercised; he would choose the one who exercised. Of course, we know that it is better to do both. Exercise is extremely important to the health and healing of the body. It helps to "pump" out toxins and poisons.

The type of exercise is also important. In order for exercise to be the most beneficial for the heart and lungs it needs to be aerobic. Aerobic exercises are those that are:

1. Continuous
2. Rhythmic
3. Use the large muscles of the body. (legs and hips)

Some of the exercises that fit into this category are: swimming, jogging, jogger-walking, walking, bicycling, jump-roping, mini-trampoline jogging and jumping, and aerobic dancing.

Aerobic exercise strengthens the cardiovascular system and the legs, which act as an auxiliary pump for the cardiovascular system. The heart is made to beat faster, putting out more oxygen-carrying blood to the cells and taking away more impurities from them. The increased oxygenization of the cells and thus the body, along with the faster removal of impurities and carbon dioxide is one of the reasons people feel more *energy* if they exercise. The body also learns to use more oxygen and yet use it more efficiently. Aerobic exercise is good for the lungs and helps calcium retention in the body. It also builds co-ordination and balance.

# MINI-TRAMPOLINE EXERCISE

Jumping on a mini-trampoline or "rebounding," as it is sometimes called, is an exercise that has all of the benefits of aerobic exercise plus more. It causes less stress on the skeletal system because the trampoline takes most of the stress. It tones and strengthens every cell in the body, cleanses the entire system of toxins and poisons, and uses the force of gravity in an acceleration/deceleration effect in the body.

The majority of people including the elderly, blind, physically and mentally handicapped, babies, and even people in wheelchairs are able to use a mini-trampoline. A baby can be held while someone is jumping, people in wheelchairs can put their feet on the trampoline while someone else jumps.

### Tones and Strengthens every cell

Rebounding exercise increases the gravitational pull on the body. At the top of the bounce the body becomes weightless for a split second. At the bottom of the bounce the body receives as much as 2 G's force. This increased pull causes the cells to tone and strengthen themselves. Bones become more dense, all muscles organs and tissues become stronger.

### Acceleration/Deceleration Cleansing Effect

The Lymphatic System of the body has 3 times more fluid than blood. It is called the vacuum cleaner or garbage collector of the body. It also is the immune system of the body. This fluid (the same fluid that fills blisters) bathes the cells in nutrients. It flows through the body in a system of tubes with one way valves. Dr. Corwin West claims trapped protein gets in the valves and that rebounding is the best way to circulate the Lymphatic System.

The bottom of the bounce causes increased pressure and closes the valves. In the middle of the bounce the valves open and at the height or top of the bounce the fluids begin to flow. As the body descends (deceleration) the fluid flows pulling waste matter away from the cells to be eliminated by lymph fluids. All cells in the body are helped by this cleaning process.

CHAPTER **13**

# *Positive Power*

## POSITIVE POWER

### What you think you are, you are.

The human brain is marvelous and complex. The mind has been compared to a robot; what you tell it, it believes. We can learn to use this "robot" of the brain rather than have it use us. Positive thoughts can actually become a power to change our lives and our health.

Many great athletes are noted for their ability to stay mentally "on top". They refuse to allow negative thinking to interfere with their game or their ability. They use positive "self-talk" to keep from downgrading themselves. We also can learn to use positive "self-talk" to lift ourselves. It is just as easy to learn to say "I want to be on time" as it is "I don't want to be late". We can learn to say to ourselves "I don't know how to do _____, but I can learn," rather than "I can't do anything, I'm not worth anything". Every person on this earth is an example of an intricate, wonderful design, we have no right to downgrade ourselves or others. But we can appreciate the wonders of life and our opportunities to live it.

What you think actually affects your health. Those people who believe they will become sick usually have their expectations fulfilled, and those who say they rarely get sick also have their expectations fulfilled. It has been found very important for cancer patients to keep a positive attitude and positive thoughts to help fight the disease. It is interesting to note that when we are sick, we are often depressed and out-of-sorts. Perhaps we should consider happiness and positive thinking as a weapon against disease.

To those who are sick or depressed now, it may be easy to read about being positive but hard to practice. Part of your responsibility is to try to eliminate the cause of your illness and depression. Other chapters in this book have been written to give aid with your physical body. Most people are able to improve but others, because of past injuries or genetic inheritance, may never be completely well. Even for these few, life does not need to be unhappy. Many lessons in gratitude, cheerfulness, and happiness are taught to the world by those who seem to be unfortunate. A positive attitude, a cheery disposition, a welcoming smile are among the greatest possessions in the world. These possessions are within the grasp of anyone who seeks them.

How do we seek them? First, know that it is possible to have them. Second, realize that each of us is responsible for our own happiness. We cannot blame any person or thing for our unhappiness. All of us have trials and troubles, that is the way of life. Some of those trials and troubles are very hard indeed, but we can make it through. (Much talking to our Maker helps make the path easier. And to those who see another going through a crisis or troubled time, it is good to have an understanding heart, a listening ear, a helping hand, and a non-gossiping mouth.) Sometimes remembering that "this too will pass" and become a memory, helps in the time of deep trials. But to those who are simply looking for a scapegoat for their unhappy lives it is time to know that the responsibility for your life and happiness rests with you.

As we grow older our bodies become worn out (some of us wear our bodies out sooner than we need to by improper habits) and we eventually die and return to our maker. This is the natural order of things, but that doesn't mean that the journey is a depressing or unhappy one. Trials and troubles do not mean that all of our life needs to be unhappy. The only person who can make you happy is you. It is up to you to decide how you want to live your life—as a happy person or as an unhappy one. It depends upon you and your attitude. Circumstances do not control your happiness. You do. And you **can**.

Suggested Reading:
1. The Holy Scriptures
2. Books or tapes by Denis E. Waitley
3. Books or tapes by Zig Zigler
4. *Man's Search For Meaning*, by Viktor E. Frankl
5. There are many many books written to help develop positive thinking habits. Read many to give yourself something good to think about.

# BIBLIOGRAPHY

Ashmead, DeWayne Ph.D. "Chelated Minerals—An Essential Component of Life".

Airola, Paavo. *How To Get Well*. Health Plus Publishers, 1974.

Airola, Paavo. "Garlic: Poison or Miracle Food?". *Let's Live*, November 1977, Volume 45, Number 11. Los Angeles, California: Oxford Industries, Inc.

Burnett and Weis. *Colon Cleanse*. Copyright pending.

Burroughs, Stanley. *The Master Cleanser*. Stanley Burroughs, 1976.

Carter, Albert E. *The Miracles of Rebound Exercise*. The National Institute of Reboundology and Health, Inc. Edmonds, Washington, 1980.

Cooper, K.H. *Aerobics*. New York: M. Evans and Co. Inc., 1968.

Crain, Lloyd. *Magic Vitamins and Organic Foods*. Crandrich Studios, Los Angeles, California, 1971.

Davis, Adelle. *Let's Get Well*. Harcourt, Brace, and World., New York, 1965,

Dickey, Esther. *Passport to Survival*. Bookcraft Publishers, Salt Lake City, Utah, 1969.

Duke, James A. Ph.D. *CRC Handbook of Medicinal Herbs*. CRC Press, Inc. Boca Raton, Florida, 1985.

Faelten, Sharon. *The Complete Book of Minerals for Health*. Rodale Press, 1981.

Gray, Robert. *The Colon Health Book*. Rockbridge Publishing Company, Oakland, California, 1980.

Griffin, La Dean. *Is Any Sick Among You?*. BiWorld Publishers, Provo, Utah, 1974.

Hansen, Maurice. *Cider Vinegar*. Arco Publishing Inc., New York, New York, 1974.

Heckman, Richard A. Ph.D. and Noorlander, Daniel O. "The Bacteriocidal Properties of Comfrey, (*Symphytum officinale*) Herbal Extracts", World Dairy and Food Research Associates, Patent Pending.

Heinerman, John. *Science of Herbal Medicine*. BiWorld Publishers, Orem, Utah, 1973.

Hills, Christopher. *The Secrets of Spirulina*. University of the Trees Press, Boulder Creek, California, 1980.

Hirsch, Roseann. "Acidophilus; What is it?"

Hogle, Mary C. *Foods That Alkalinize and Heal*. Health Research, Mokelumme, California.

Jensen, Bernard. *Health Magic Through Chlorophyll from Living Plant Life*. BiWorld Publishers, Provo, Utah, 1973.

Kloss, Jethro. *Back to Eden*. Longview Pub. House, Coalmont, Tennessee, 1939.

Larsen, Gena. *Better Food for Better Babies and Their Families*. Keats Publishing Co., New Canaan, Conn.

Levit, Beverly. "Garlic, Fact and Fable."

Lust, John. *The Herb Book*. Bantam Books, Inc., 666 Fifth Avenue, New York, New York 10019.

Malstrom, Stan. *Own Your Own Body*. Fresh Mountain Air Publishing Company, 1977.

Manning, Betsy Russell. *Wheatgrass Juice*. Calistoga, Calif., 1979.

Mindell, Earl. *Vitamin Bible*. Rawson, Wade Publishers, Inc., 1979.

Moulton, Le Arta. "Nature's Medicine Chest". The Gluten Co.

Noorlander, Daniel O., "A Modern Way to Fight Infections".

Noorlander, Daniel O. and Heckman, Richard A., Ph.D., "Comfrey Herbal Extracts for Human and Veterinarian Medicine".

Noorlander, Daniel O. and Heckman, Richard A., Ph.D., "Bacteriositic Properties of Comfrey Herbal Extract. Research and Application", Patents Pending.

Nutritional Consulting Services, Inc., *Herbal Combinations, Physicians Desk Reference Manual*, Nutritional Consulting Services, Inc., Sandy, Utah, 1980.

Price, Sandy. *Fitness and Energy through Exercises*. Nature's Sunshine Products, 1978.

Reynolds, Bruford Scott. *How To Grow and Serve Sprouts*. The Reynolds Enterprise, Orangeville, Utah, 1970.

Ritchason, Jack. *The Little Herb Encyclopedia*, BiWorld Publishers, Orem, Utah, 1982.

Rosenburg, Harold Dr. with Feldzamen, A.N., Ph.D., *The Book of Vitamin Therapy*., Berkley Publishing Corporation, New York, New York 10016, 1975.

Staff of Prevention Magazine, *The Complete Book of Vitamins*, Rodale Press, Emmaus, Pennsylvania.

Tenney, Louise. *Today's Herbal Health*. Hawthorne Books, Provo, Utah, 1982.

Walker, Norman W., *Colon Health*. O'Sullivan Woodside and Co., Phoenix, Arizona, 1979.

Wigmore, Ann. *Be Your Own Doctor*, Hemisphere Press, Inc.

Wright, Jonathan. *Dr. Wright's Book of Nutritional Therapy*, Rodale Press, Inc., Emmaus, Pennsylvania, 1982.

# INDEX

**249**